ODD
GIRL
SPEAKS
OUT

RACHEL SIMMONS

ODD GIRL SPEAKS OUT

GIRLS WRITE ABOUT BULLIES, CLIQUES, POPULARITY, AND JEALOUSY

A HARVEST ORIGINAL
HARCOURT, INC.
Orlando   Austin   New York   San Diego   Toronto   London

For information about permission to reproduce
selections from this book, write to Permissions,
Houghton Mifflin Harcourt Publishing Company,
215 Park Avenue South, New York, New York 10003.

www.hmhbooks.com

Library of Congress Cataloging-in-Publication Data
Odd girl speaks out: girls write about bullies, cliques, popularity,
and jealousy/Rachel Simmons, [editor].—1st ed.
p. cm.
ISBN 0-15-602815-8
ISBN 978-0-15602-815-8
1. Girls—Psychology.   2. Interpersonal relations in children.
3. Interpersonal conflict in children.   4. Aggressiveness in children.
5. Bullying.   6. Cliques (Sociology).
I. Simmons, Rachel, 1966–
HQ777.O33   2004
305.23'082--dc22   2003020672

Text set in Sabon
Designed by Linda Lockowitz

Printed in the United States of America
First edition
DOC 10 9 8 7 6 5

Harcourt Trade Publishers books may be purchased for educational,
business, or sales promotional use. For information please write:
Harcourt Trade Publishers, attn: Director of Special Sales,
525 B Street, Suite 1900, San Diego, CA 92101.

CONTENTS

A NOTE FROM RACHEL SIMMONS

Did you read *Odd Girl Out*? Got a story about girls that you want to tell? Want to get your story published?" I asked girls for their stories with a flyer bearing this invitation. I mailed and e-mailed the flyer hundreds of times, handed it out at my book signings and speeches all over the country, and posted it on my Web site to be downloaded. I received hundreds of e-mails and letters, and even a CD from an aspiring young songwriter. The Internet sent my flyer so far that letters came from England, Canada, and Australia.

As an editor, my priority was to preserve the girls' voices and stories. I edited their work for spelling and length, and I changed some story titles to give readers a better idea of the content; where girls did not provide a title, I supplied one.

Parents and guardians submitted written permission for the authors to publish stories in this book. To protect everyone involved, however, I have made some changes. None of the authors are identified by their names. I have changed the names of other individuals mentioned in the stories. Finally, I have omitted or altered the names of screen names, cities, and schools.

A month before I finished *Odd Girl Speaks Out,* I received an e-mail from a seventh-grade girl warning me that one of my authors had omitted some crucial facts. In her piece, "Kendra" wrote that she was victimized without warning by several friends. Those friends, the e-mailer wrote, had good reason to do this.

She explained that as recently as that day, Kendra had become angry and spread several vicious rumors about her. There are, the anonymous writer concluded, two sides to every story.

The stories are published here in order to provide a public space for girls to discuss a part of their lives that is often silenced. Yet we would all do well to heed this middle schooler's advice. Every girl writes from her own vantage point, and circumstances often conspire to muddy girls' perspectives on their conflicts. For example, when girls struggle to communicate why they're angry, their target may not know why she is being hurt. Please keep in mind that the authors' opinions are not intended as the last word on any incident, only as a snapshot of their lives.

I invite readers' feedback. Please visit my Web site, www.rachelsimmons.com, to share your comments.

THE SOUND OF A GIRL'S VOICE

Introduction

I was worried about Emma. She'd been at my girls' leadership camp for three days and had barely spoken. She was twelve, with dark hair and soft, downcast eyes. Even though she sat with the other girls at meals, I couldn't tell if she was really making friends. She was short and quiet and easily invisible.

One afternoon, I led a lively discussion about bullying among girls. A few hours later, after swimming, there was a knock at my door. It was Emma. Delighted, I started to welcome her, and before I could finish my sentence she was telling me a story, something she had kept so secret she was afraid that even to greet me might change her mind.

It was Valentine's Day in fifth grade, and Emma had driven her best friends crazy with her crush on Zack. She hoped he knew how she felt, prayed for a card from him, doodled his name inside her notebook.

It was also the day after her best friend sat their clique in a circle at lunchtime and gave them each a grade out of one hundred. It was a weekly ritual that Emma anticipated with a mixture of dread and hope. Each time, she hoped she would make it out of the sixties and into C range. Yesterday, she'd gotten a fifty-nine, a point below passing.

Today, when she went to her locker during social studies, the curling, shiny red paper was there, protruding out of the locker door. Slowly, she opened the card. "Dear Emma," it read, "I love the way your fat spills over your jeans when you wear those tight shirts. Will you be my valentine? Love, Zack."

She looked out my window, then back at me.

"I can't stop thinking of that image, over and over again," she told me. Emma had been making herself throw up ever since.

I began consoling her frantically, but she only nodded. I wasn't entirely sure she could hear me. By dinner, I knew it didn't matter. Emma was talking and laughing with the other seventh grade girls. The next day, she began raising her hand in discussions. When it was time for the girls to run their own discussions, Emma convinced her group to return to the topic of girl bullying. She served as the moderator. Then, standing before more than thirty people, Emma told the other girls exactly what had happened to her.

To write *Odd Girl Out,* I met with hundreds of girls in groups. We'd sit on the floor in a circle, cross-legged and munching snacks. I figured girls would be more comfortable talking together about bullying, meanness, and conflict. I thought they talked about it all the time.

I was wrong. When I asked them questions about direct confrontation, there was silence. A hand crept into the air, and a girl confided her fear of losing friends. Another confessed she might say something she didn't mean. The others stared at her, hesitated, then raised their hands and started talking. Whispers skittered through the room.

It soon became clear that most girls thought they were the only ones afraid of losing friends, the only ones who felt like their world might end if they did, the only ones with secrets about being bullies and victims, with knots in their stomachs as they entered the cafeteria and wondered where to sit.

As their voices grew more confident, their relief was palpable. They hadn't talked about this at all, and it thrilled them to realize they weren't alone. Sitting with the girls, watching them watch each other, was one of the most exciting parts of the *Odd Girl Out* project.

I invited young writers to tell their stories of bullying and friendship because I wanted girls to talk directly to each other about the hidden culture of aggression. I wanted to give every girl a chance to be a part of those discussion circles.

In *Odd Girl Out,* I explored how our culture affects the ways girls show their anger. Through powerful messages sent by parents, teachers, friends, and the media, girls learn that anger will not be tolerated; that they must sit quietly and behave like perfect little angels; that they cannot be ugly to anyone; and that breaking any of these rules will bring swift, severe punishment.

But much as girls try, bad feelings can't be wished or forced away. As a result, many girls hide their anger, using body language (the silent treatment), relationships (ganging up and threatening not to be friends with someone), and indirect aggression (rumors, gossip, the Internet) to express their true feelings. Others stifle their feelings, becoming depressed, cutting themselves, or developing eating disorders.

When girls are mean to each other, most people shrug it off. Determined to keep its girls "sugar and spice and everything nice," society turns a blind eye to girls' aggression. "Girls will be girls," they say. Or, they cluck, "It's a phase all girls go through."

As a result, most girls suffer alone. Their situations aren't addressed, their pain is private, and their problems hidden. Now, that's changing. We're starting to think about what girls do as "aggression," not just a "rite of passage." *Odd Girl Out* and Rosalind Wiseman's *Queen Bees and Wannabees* began building a public consciousness of what it means to be hurt in social, relational, or indirect ways.

We must continue that process, this time in girls' voices. Girls need to tell their own stories, to each other and to the world. This book is intended not only to help girls but also to be a powerful declaration, a kind of petition signed by girls.

My strongest memory of being bullied as a third grader was the feeling that no one had ever gone through what I had. If that was true, then it also was true that I was a loser of epic proportions, and that what happened was clearly my fault. Those feelings of responsibility marked me deeply. They had a huge impact on my self-esteem. I know I ended up writing *Odd Girl Out* because of them.

But I hadn't just been a victim. I did something terrible to a close friend when I was fourteen. As the years passed, I buried the memory deep inside my mind. I lied to myself and others about who I was, convinced I had never been anything but nice. Later in the book, I'll explore how hiding a real, human part of my personality damaged my ability to have healthy conflicts with my friends and nearly denied Anne the dignity of an apology.

When you realize the confusion, panic, pain, hurt, and anger you experienced is something that millions of other girls have gone through, it changes things. First of all, it's a lot harder to blame yourself as a victim. Second, when you understand your situation and see it as something relatively common, it gives you a context for your pain, not to mention some perspective. Finally, if you were a bully, understanding that aggression is normal can help you take responsibility for your actions and grow as a person in significant ways.

Telling her story freed Emma from silence and shame. It gave her back some of the joys of girlhood that had been taken from her. I know I can't erase the searing loneliness of being an odd girl out. Yet I hope this book will give girls a sense of community, an opportunity to share strategies and solace, and most of all, the knowledge that even the worst kind of heartbreak improves with time.

What Girls Do

A shake of the head, a roll of the eyes
The rumors the lies
They no longer play on your pride
But rip you up inside
This is what girls do
This is what they say
It is like this every day
The mothers reply
But that is a lie
Walking in the hall
Taking in it all
All alone no one home
Kids shouting, kids staring
All this torture I'm bearing
No one caring

—AGE 12

Growing from the Pain

Grammar school is where aggression all began for me. I went to a little Catholic private school, in a little "dandy" town in New Jersey. Everyone was friends with everyone else; it was hard not to be, in a class of thirty-five! But even that had its downfalls.

It all started in the sixth grade when little groups and cliques of girls formed. I seemed to fit in with everyone, not because I was popular but because I was always the "nice girl." I won "nicest" in the yearbook and "most Christianlike" at church. But even being nice had its downfalls. People could easily take advantage of you and in my case this one girl, Alisa, somehow became my nightmare.

It all began when she started to become best friends with all my friends. I loved it at first because it became one "happy group" but little by little I noticed Alisa slowly acting differently toward me. Then the stories started. Lie after lie, rumor after rumor was created as I sat there in awe of why and what she was trying to do to me. It just didn't make sense. Another problem I had was that I was very shy and hardly stood up for myself because even when I tried, Alisa would often "shut me down" and turn things around once again.

My life seemed to be a bad dream playing over and over again in my mind. "Poor Alisa" tried to turn things around and accused me of doing what she had done to me (which of course never happened). Then eighth grade graduation came. I thought I would finally be able to get away from the misery I was put through.

I remember sitting at home crying for hours, thinking how she got away with all she put me through and why she tried to make my life so miserable. Even when I went to my best friends for advice (which were also her best friends, conveniently), they would just say that they didn't want to get involved because no one wanted to get tied up in "Alisa's lies." Half of them had been there and no one wanted to go through it time after time.

I finally thought when high school came along it would end! But of course it didn't. Alisa followed me right to high school along with ten other girls from my old school. I made a promise to myself at that point that I wouldn't let her bring me down. This was my time to shine. My high school years were going to be memorable and I was going to be out there making friends, making memories, and making a future that no one, especially Alisa, was going to stop me from having.

The first few months were hell as she tried to hold on to every last strand of me she could. She began to realize that I didn't need to get caught in her little games anymore. I began to meet new people and make new friendships, and Alisa got jealous. Alisa was finally getting a taste of what I had always hoped for: the realization that she couldn't rule me anymore.

Months passed and our paths crossed but I kept my distance and watched what I said. I even began to feel bad for her because I learned what fueled her popularity. It was her meanness, and the only way she thrived was through it. I learned that the only reason she was popular was not because she was smart or nice or athletic or pretty (the so-called ideal popular girl), but because she was cruel. The reason people wanted to be her friend was to avoid confrontation.

I sit back now in amazement of why and how I let things get to the point they did; how I allowed someone to take over my life as she did. I do thank Alisa, though, because she showed me someone I would never want to be. I now treat my relationships very differently. I *think* before I say something dehumanizing or negative.

Even Alisa has changed. As my senior year comes to an end, I can say that Alisa and I are better now. We occasionally hang out with the same people and even talk now. Alisa seemed to grow out of her meanness, and I guess you could say I grew out of my vulnerable niceness.

Sometimes a person's only way to express their hurtful feelings inside is by trashing it all on someone else. It was very unfortunate for Alisa to leave me with negative memories of our grammar school years together, but it is uplifting to feel that in the end everything turned out okay. Without Alisa in my life, I wouldn't have grown into the individual I am today.

—AGE 18

I Don't Know Where I Stand

I "flapped" my hand over the small square of paper. Hands sweating, face red, throat dry.

"What could I have possibly done?" I thought. My head felt dizzy and heavy. My eyes tight. Jaw clenched.

I pulled the square truth out of my pocket. My hands were sweating and the back of my neck felt tight.

One, two, three. I opened the first fold. My stomach knotted. I opened the entire thing. Skimmed it enough to get the idea of the whole thing. It wasn't as bad as I thought it was going to be. I skimmed it once more and refolded it into my pocket. Now my hands were shaking.

I had found out why. Why Sophie didn't invite me to her party.

It all started on a Monday, during lunch.

"So what do you want for your birthday?" Those were the words that started it all.

I knew Sophie's birthday was soon. But I didn't

know if the words meant there was a party or there would be a party.

The next day I asked one of the people I knew Sophie would invite if Sophie was having a party.

"Yeah, this Saturday."

I was hurt. I was shocked. How could Sophie invite two out of the three people she eats lunch with every day?

I thought we were friends. I thought that because we went out to lunch every day we were friends. But I guess she didn't.

The next day I asked Ava if she was going to Sophie's birthday party, half expecting her to say, "Yeah, are you?" and half expecting her to blurt out a secret Sophie told her to keep.

Instead her face turned pale and "innocent-looking."

"Yeah," she said, biting her lip, as if Sophie had told her to keep a secret from me.

The next day, instead of eating with Sophie and her "birthday crew" I ate with Ramona, a friend I knew I could trust. We sat at a table right behind Sophie and her birthday crew, whispering about how they hardly noticed I was gone.

A few days later I asked one of Sophie's birthday crew why Sophie didn't invite me.

He looked as if Sophie had said something really nasty about me.

"Wait, just tell me a little bit," I said, with fear that I would start crying wildly.

"It's something in your personality that she doesn't like. And her mom doesn't like you for that, either."

What could I have possibly done to make Sophie's *mom* not like me? I don't even know Sophie's mom!

Finally at the last period on Friday I asked one of the birthday crew to write down why Sophie hadn't invited me. I opened the paper, which would reveal the truth. It read:

> Sophie didn't invite you because she thinks you'll steal all the attention away from her and control the party. She also thinks you act like you're the only one who's allowed to be friends with Ava. This is the same reason Sophie's mom doesn't like you.

First of all, the guests would come to see her, not me. And secondly, I can't "control" the party. It's her party. And I'm the only one who's "allowed" to be friends with Ava? Ava's allowed to be friends with whoever she wants. I do admit I sometimes (sort of) hog her, but hardly ever.

The Monday after the party I asked a birthday crew member how the party was.

"Good."

"What did you do?" I asked.

"Talked, watched movies."

"What did you talk about?"

"Stuff."

"Me?"

"Um, no."

"Yes, you did!"

"No."

"Come on, you're lying," I said, not really knowing I cracked something open.

"Well, yeah."

"What did you say about me?"

"Sophie asked why you were upset."

"And what did you say?"

"I said you thought you didn't do those things all the time."

"And what did she say?"

"She agreed."

After all that! After all that she put me through. After the worrying and the putting the pieces together she agreed that I don't (always) do the things she said I did. I still wonder if she's sorry she didn't include me in the party.

I still have friendship problems with Sophie and Ava. They leave me out or talk behind my back. Especially Sophie. I don't know where I stand with them. Part of me wants to be all "friendly" and doing everything together, but part of me doesn't. It will take a long time before I can ever even consider forgiving Sophie (or Ava).

—AGE 13

They Weren't There Anymore

I've always been the odd one out
In almost everything.
I've never found a crowd that I've actually belonged to.
So therefore
I'm left out of a lot of things.
I'm even left out of things
When it comes to my own family,
My cousins.

I've already gotten used to
Not being told anything
(such as secrets)
and being excluded
from many things.
But I wanted
To be a part of this
Badly.
My cousins were planning
To go to Skate-key
(a skating rink)

and I love
anything having to do with
dancing or skating
So I asked
If I could go with them
And they said
Sure.
I then went
To go get my skates
And when I returned
They weren't there anymore.

By then
I was already used to it,
So I wasn't so hurt.
Instead
I just sat down and watched TV
And read a book.
Then I ate food.
And waited
Until they came back at around seven p.m.
And stared at them all
For at least five minutes
And
Left.

—AGE 12

Strengthened Spirit

It is funny how in all the days, weeks, and years in our lifetimes that flee before our eyes, certain memories cannot evade our grasp and continue to live on in our hearts forever. Sometimes it takes the wounded heart years to heal from the inflicted pain, but for some, those scars can leave a permanent mark than can never be erased. I can still feel fierce twinges of pain when I reflect upon my experiences in a friendship that I had in years past. For a while, I tried to forget, but once you have been cut as deeply as I have, the pain cannot just dissipate, for it has been branded into my heart, and will forever continue to leave a lasting impact on my life.

I was just a mere sixth grader, both innocent and naive as I tried to blend in with the rest of the girls in my tight-knit elementary school. At first, I felt content with my group of friends, for although I was not the leader, I was still surrounded by peers, and I was willing to follow along if it guaranteed acceptance. I never anticipated that these girls who I considered friends would make my life a living hell for an entire year. I was very trusting and honestly believed that my friends were good people as well.

The onset of my tarnished friendship started out small, as my group did little things outside of school and failed to invite me along. This caused me some pain, but I tried to have faith that they would include me next time. Soon, it became a regular occurrence, and to make matters worse, I would have to sit in class and listen to them talking about funny stories from the times they had spent together. The only reason I subjected myself to this torment was because when I was with any one of my friends *alone,* she would treat me like a true friend would.

To compensate for my feelings of loneliness and isolation, I tried to include myself into their conversations and act interested in their stories so that I would be included, too. Even when they did include me in their activities, I still felt left out, because they would all stick together and make me feel like an outsider. That year, my sole ambition was to be recognized and accepted by my friends because, more than anything else, I longed for their affection.

Before I knew it, my group of friends started to become more devious and malicious, and I began to realize that their inside jokes were mainly based on poking fun at me. No matter what I did, they always found a way to make me feel embarrassed, whether it was something that I said or even the way I played a sport. The secretive gossip made me feel awful, and I'll admit they succeeded in taking away a great deal of my self-esteem. Soon, I caught onto more and more of the little subliminal messages in their conversation. They got much entertainment out of paining me and literally tearing me apart.

Perhaps it was because I was a good student, or because I was a kind, unassuming person, but for whatever reason, I became the victim of the group. Because of this false sense of camaraderie, I allowed myself to believe that they really did want me as a friend. If only I had known that deep down they were just using me as a scapegoat to lash out all of their insecurities on, then maybe I could have saved myself a lot sooner.

Because it was virtually four against one, I felt helpless. I had no allies to back me up, so I continued to play the role of the victim. If I would've had one person to back me up, I would have felt stronger and more assertive. I knew that if I tried to fight back, I would just be further ridiculed. As the months of verbal abuse went on, I would come home from school each day in tears and cry to my mother about how horribly I was being treated. Both of my parents assured me that the girls were just jealous of me, and that they had to make fun of me to make themselves feel better. My parents always told me to remember that I was a better person, and that one day I would find real friends. To me, that day seemed like it would never come.

As the year progressed, I began to dread going to

school. I knew that they were making a mockery out of me and the emotional pain was more than I could bear. No matter what I did, my friends would find a way to turn it against me and use it as fuel for their own personal jokes. It got to the point where I even quit baton twirling. Baton was something that I genuinely liked, but my insecurities forced me to quit. I knew that their eyes were on me at all times, just waiting for me to make a mistake so they could use it against me the next day. Back then I didn't realize it, but they were just trying to put me down so that they could feel more powerful. I was too timid to confront them.

Eventually, all of the months of my agony and crying to my parents boiled up to a climax. I was just checking my mail on the Internet one day, and I came across a letter from one of my male friends that said, "I found this e-mail going around, and I thought you ought to see it." To my dismay, this e-mail was entirely devoted to destroying my reputation and making me look like a complete loser. The e-mail was harsh, cruel, humiliating, insulting, and degrading. It was during this moment that I had an epiphany.

I knew that I had let the abuse go on long enough, and I was not going to take it anymore. Although I cried hysterically upon reading the e-mail, I decided to show it to my mother, who was utterly horrified by its contents. My mom was enraged that anyone would stoop low enough to degrade someone behind their back, just for sheer enjoyment, so she retaliated by e-mailing the author of the vicious e-mail back a little letter of her own that sought to put the girl in her place.

I was so happy that I was getting my justice because one of my friends had finally been caught in the act and was about to be punished. I don't know if I ever thanked the boy who showed me the e-mail enough. Whether he knew it or not, his courage and sense of justice changed my life that year. Thanks to this boy, my friends finally got what they deserved. Now, they had my mom against them and they no longer had me as a friend.

By the end of that school year, I learned a lot about myself and just how strong I really was without them. I was extremely proud of myself for standing up to my ex-friends. I proved that my internal strength was more potent than any of their harmful words. Although I successfully escaped from the friendship nightmare and found replacement friends, I still felt the emotional repercussions.

For the rest of elementary school, I felt insecure about my new friends because I was afraid that they would betray me and stab me in the back like my former friends did. It was hard for me to trust even my closest friends, because I had been wounded so severely by my last painful experience, but eventually the tides turned.

Now, as a junior in high school, I have moved on and found a close group of friends that has made my life seem more complete. I feel as though I have gotten my justice, because now I am the one with genuine, loyal, trustworthy friends who I can rely on for anything, while my former friends drifted apart and became sort of lost.

In a funny way, my harsh experience has liberated me. It gave me character and enough courage to stand up for what I believe in. I will never allow myself to become a victim as long as I live.

I have learned that sometimes negative experiences can have positive outcomes. They provide us with the courage to go on through adversity and equip us with strength and perseverance.

In a way I am thankful that I was faced with such a negative situation because the same girls who sought to destroy my spirit actually succeeded in making me the empowered person that I am today. Although I will always harbor memories of that painful time in my heart, I can walk taller each day knowing that I am stronger because of it. *No one* can ever take that away from me.

—AGE 17

Quality, Not Quantity

Growing up in a small town where everyone knows everyone, cliques are formed early in elementary school and are often a bit catty and almost cultlike. You are taught by the "leaders" (often the prettiest or the most powerful of the group) what is considered pretty, nice, and even acceptable. As a young girl, I wanted more than anything to fit in and be part of this group because everyone seemed to like these girls. I wanted to be invited to their sleepovers and laugh with them in school about the silly things that had happened there.

If you were not in their group, the girls made fun of you, yelled things at you, teased you about the way you wore your hair or the clothing you had on. In an attempt to be pretty and fit in, I developed an eating disorder. In sixth grade, my desire to be popular had fueled a full-fledged problem that has since been diagnosed as anorexia.

During middle school I continued to be friends with these girls, scared of what would happen if I decided to leave their group for people who were more like me. At a gathering one day, I happened to kiss a boy that one of my friends had a crush on. By the next day, it was all over school and Emily, my friend who had the crush, had ordered all of the other girls not to talk to me. They made a Web page about me that said mean, untrue things, such as that I was a lesbian, that I had had sex with at least twenty guys, and that I was pregnant. These statements were damaging to my reputation as well as to my self-confidence. As I walked down the halls at school, the girls would scream "SLUT," "WHORE," and many other hurtful words that shouldn't be used against anyone, regardless of their age. I had Snapple bottles thrown at my head and I was forced to eat lunch in the bathroom by myself, embarrassed and unsure of what to do.

I went home every day and cried, begging my mom to let me switch schools. My mother dismissed the problems as "girls being girls" and figured that as we neared high school the girls would grow out of this "phase" and become more mature. They didn't. The name-calling and slandering and spreading of rumors went on as my eating disorder grew progressively worse. I had no one to turn to. My mother was my only friend.

At last my mother realized the seriousness of the situation and allowed me to transfer to a Catholic school my junior year. Everyone told me that I would make friends quickly because of my outgoing personality, but I was worried that everyone would already have cliques and that I would be an outsider. On my first day of school a girl whom I'll call Gossip befriended me. She introduced me to all her friends and took me in. I felt wanted and needed and liked, things I hadn't felt in a very long time.

Not too soon after, I noticed that Gossip was very powerful in the school. Everyone was terrified of her because she spoke her mind and made fun of everyone. NO one wanted to be on her bad side. She was always jealous of my weight and wanted to be as thin as me, not knowing I had to starve myself to be this way. One day she decided to let jealousy rear its ugly head, and she proceeded to turn every girl in my grade against me. I thought that girls were supposed to grow out of this.

Gossip and the rest of my friends wouldn't look at me. They would still yell things at me down the halls like "anorexic bitch," and Gossip threatened to punch my face in. I came into school one day and there were pictures taped to my locker of my friends and I with my face cut out. I got so upset that I was diagnosed with clinical depression and put on Prozac — as if that would make the girls like me again.

Eventually the girls got over it and found someone new to pick on. I, however, was scarred for life. Terrified to trust anyone, I kept all my feelings inside, and walked on eggshells around everyone, careful not to say a word that might offend anyone.

The summer going into my senior year I realized a few things. I realized that I liked who I was as a person, and that was all that mattered. I had a few close friends who had never betrayed me, and I focused on further improving my relationships with them. I took comfort in the fact that I had a loving family. Last, I learned to voice my opinions and to speak up for myself.

I was a new person my senior year and everyone knew it. Although I was still the same sweet girl who had been hurt many times before, I was stronger because of everything that had happened, and my eyes showed it. People respected me. As I prepare to go off to college, I know I will probably only keep in touch with a few people from high school. But I have learned that with friendship, it's quality, not quantity. If you learn to respect yourself, others will follow. I've learned to live by the quote, "Be yourself and you will find, who minds doesn't matter and who matters won't mind."

—AGE 17

"WHY IS IT MY FAULT THAT I DON'T WANT TO BE HER FRIEND?"
Moving On, Growing Apart

In this section, girls write from both sides about the uncomfortable moment when friends start to grow apart. Of all the problems girls face in their friendships, this is one of the hardest. One girl feels she is being cruelly abandoned, even bullied. The other girl thinks she shouldn't have to be close to someone she just doesn't feel the same way about anymore. There is silence and denial on one side, and desperation and panic on the other.

We live in a culture that tells girls to be friends with everyone. There is a language and even an industry to support best friendships between two girls: "BFF" and broken heart necklaces come quickly to mind. But what happens when that changes? We know that guys and girls break up; we accept that without question. We probably have more books on how to deal with that than about how to end poverty.

Yet best friends can be just as close as a romantic couple, and we have no idea how to confront changes in the relationship, or to break up. No one prepares us for it, tells us how to do it, or what to expect. No one says it's okay, or not. As a result, people call it bullying. Others are outraged that they're being called bullies. Adults take their cues from the girls but don't know much more.

Here are girls' perspectives on outgrowing a friendship, along with some suggestions on how to deal with it.

Why Is It My Fault That
I Don't Want to Be Her Friend?

It was freshman year of high school at an all-girls' school, and Maya was in my math class. It was honors algebra. She was also in my homeroom. I thought she was so cool. She had these bright pink shoelaces, and she had this aura of confidence about her. A couple of months into the school year we started to hang out.

We always had fun together. We would hang out at the local theme park, go to the mall, or just spend the night at each others' houses. But it wasn't just the two of us. Two friends from my old school also hung out with us. Ellie, one of them, didn't like Maya. I knew this, but to be nice, she would still hang out with us. Jenny, my other friend, became superclose with Maya also, which I didn't mind because it made it easy for the three of us to hang out.

After a few months, I started to notice negative changes in my personality. You see, Maya was an only child and was used to a lot of attention. She was slightly on the selfish side but I didn't really mind. I am the youngest of three children, and by default given a lot of attention myself. I found myself competing with Maya for attention. This brought out a lot of selfish tendencies in me. When I began to notice the changes in me, I knew I had to do something. I just didn't know what.

One weekend Maya invited Jenny, Ellie, and me up to her beach house for the weekend. Ellie politely declined the offer with some conveniently made-up conflict. However Jenny and I accepted; we had previously spent a weekend up there and enjoyed it.

Jenny had an appointment the day that we left, but I just went to Maya's house after school. While there, I was stuck with Maya's nostalgia. We watched what seemed to be four hours of her dance recitals. I simply couldn't take it anymore, but I kept it in because we would be together all weekend. Jenny finally arrived and we headed to the beach house.

On Saturday morning, Maya and Jenny woke up early and tried to wake me up. I was tired and told them that I wanted to sleep. They let me sleep, but while I was sleeping they went to the little shop that was my favorite, without me. When I got up they were still gone but returned shortly.

I didn't know what they did while I was asleep and didn't find out until Sunday, when I asked if we could go to that store and they said they already had while I was sleeping. I simply couldn't take it any more. I put on a good face for the rest of vacation, but knew it wouldn't last any longer. When I got home, I knew it was time to end it.

I tried to avoid conflict but really hit it head on. Monday morning I avoided talking to Maya at all costs. She just thought I wasn't feeling well. By Tuesday she knew that something was wrong. I simply told her that I didn't want to be her friend anymore.

On Wednesday she had one of my best friends on her side, Jenny. Jenny wrote I was a bitch on Maya's hand before school one morning. Ellie, who somehow remained neutral, informed me of something on Maya's hand but wouldn't tell me because she knew it would offend me.

In homeroom that day, I had a friend go and see what was written on her hand. At first she showed her clean hand. But my friend asked to see the other hand. She reported back to me and I told our homeroom teacher. Ms. Baker talked to her until the end of homeroom. When questioned about it, her only defense was that she wasn't the one who wrote it.

The next few months were long. Maya could not accept the fact that I didn't want to be her friend. This was partly my fault because I wouldn't tell her why, just that I didn't want to be her friend. Things kept escalating. Once a week we were in the counselor's office because I was affecting her grades.

I didn't understand: Why couldn't she just get over the fact that I didn't want her to be my friend? What did they think was going to happen? That we would magically make up? Besides the counselor's office, we were also in the dean's office. Everything seemed to be poor

Maya, poor Maya. Not to mention that we always had these meetings at her convenience, not mine.

I had no clue that I was being looked at as the bully. She was the one who took my best friends. She was the one who drove me to it. Why is it my fault that I don't want to be her friend? Why do I need to explain that to anyone? She always accused me of spreading rumors. Sure I was, but she was doing it just as much. Why was I the one being punished?

She was eventually able to move on and get over the fact that I didn't want to be her friend. The saddest part, however, is that my social status climbed and hers dropped. She was hanging out with the smelly cats, the kids who don't fit in socially; they're nice, but it could ruin your rep if you talk to them.

My tendencies haven't changed, I still hold everything in but I make sure that people aren't influencing me poorly. Maya, however, left our school the next year. It was reportedly because she didn't like her teachers, but everyone knew the real reason. I changed someone's life forever because I simply couldn't tell her how I felt.

Our society put me on a pedestal for it. I secretly know the truth. And I will have to live my life knowing I did that to someone. Yet I still can't understand why it is my entire fault. I was protecting myself. Am I sorry? Yes. Will I ever have the chance to tell her? Probably not.

—AGE 17

We Were Best Friends in Fifth Grade

We were best friends in fifth grade. Amy and I happened to be sitting next to each other that first day of school. Her other best friend, Camille, was in the other fifth grade class, and they still spoke often. However, Amy and I had more time together, and so our bond grew. We used to have sleepovers and watch movies and other things that little girls did. I don't go to sleepovers anymore.

Later that year, my eyesight began to worsen and I needed glasses. The first time I went over to her house, all I remember is standing in her bedroom, telling her to shut up, as she called me four eyes. The thing about Amy was that no matter how many times I told her to be quiet, she'd just keep on saying whatever she wanted, louder and louder, until it began to invade the dark corridors of my mind. After that day, I didn't wear my glasses anymore. I spent the rest of my childhood blinded to the world.

When sixth grade came, my worst fear came true.

Amy was in my class, but so was Camille. Somehow, even within my inexperienced mind, I knew it was over. Amy sat with Camille that first day of school, and every day after that. She began to exclude me from her conversations, saying, "I need to talk to Camille alone." They would end up going over to the other side of the playground, giggling. Soon enough, they just did not talk to me very much at all.

In eighth grade, we became friends again. Not exactly really good friends; I was never invited to sleepovers or parties. She was still friends with Camille, but had acquired another trooper. Melissa had transferred to our school in seventh grade. The three of them were inseparable. I don't think they went anywhere without the others. They would let me sit at their table while they ate. Sometimes they'd talk to me; sometimes they wouldn't. In ninth grade, I became closer friends with them. Once they thought I was depressed, and they gave me this basket full of goodies. I shouldn't have taken it.

That winter there was a dance. I was really excited about it, and I asked them if they were going every single day that week. They all said, "Well, no, we decided not to go." I asked them the day of the dance; I got the same reply. I called Camille up the night of the dance; she gave me the same answer. I decided not to go, either.

The next day at the bus stop, my cousin Lauren

asked me if I was at the dance last night. I told her I decided not to go because my friends hadn't. Then she
told me something that sent chills down my spine.

"But your friends were there, I saw them. They were
doing that dance. You know, the one they always practice at noon hour in the hallway?" I actually accused
her of lying to me.... This haunted the back of my
mind all that day.

That night, I decided to consult another source.
Mimi and I had spent a lot of time together the summer
before. She was always really nice to me, but I never
really fit in with her clique. I knew she'd tell me the
truth. When I got her e-mail, I shook so hard that the
keyboard rattled. She said they were there. They were
all there. "Why would they lie to you?" she said at the
end of her e-mail.

The next day at school, I cried through the morning
announcements. Mimi and her friends looked really
mad at Amy and her friends. I heard one of them say,
"That's a sin. That's mean." Amy wouldn't have it this
way, I knew she wouldn't.

"So what's wrong?" she asked me at recess.

"You guys were at the dance, you said you weren't
going. You said you didn't go the day after, even."

There was a silence.

"Well, we never wanted to hurt your feelings. We
didn't plan to go to the dance together. I wanted to go
by myself, you know, to see what would happen. I was

really disappointed when I saw Camille and Melissa there. I guess we just all decided on our own to go. What a coincidence, eh?"

What are the chances of that? I thought.

"I thought no one would ever hurt me again. I trusted you," I said, crying.

"It wasn't meant to happen," Amy said. "You should become more independent."

Melissa called me up that night, wanting to talk about what had happened.

"You shouldn't have told Mimi. Now everyone knows. Amy is really upset."

"Well, if it didn't happen that way, you shouldn't be worried. All I did was ask Mimi a simple question. She gave me an answer. Who am I supposed to talk to about my problems? Aren't I allowed to have any friends?"

"Why don't you talk to us, from now on?" Melissa replied.

The next day I didn't hang out with them. I was going to become more independent. I asked out a popular boy from school and he said yes. We became girlfriend and boyfriend. Amy must not have liked that. I hung out with him every noon hour; we would talk about how our days were while we walked around the hallways. He would give me chocolate and candy and stuffed animals and cards and letters that said *I love you.* Amy demanded to read one of them once.

"Wow, you're really lucky. This guy seems like a rare gem."

I thought my friendship with Amy was over for good. I was wrong. Later that spring, my homeroom teacher decided to change around the seating plan, leaving me sitting next to Amy. He probably thought we were still friends. So I sat by her every day. She'd always ask me if I had my homework done, and she'd peer over to check.

"Why didn't you buy any raffle tickets on the chocolate Easter bunny?" she asked me.

"I just didn't want to win it, that's all. Too much chocolate for me," I said.

"Well, you could have raffled it off again and taken the money for yourself!" she said, like it was the obvious decision. "I guess you weren't really thinking, now, were you?" I didn't know quite what to say.

"Who do you think you are? Do you think you're better than us? You're so mean and stuck up!" she said, and she did it again. She said it louder and louder and louder. I walked out of the room as my teacher walked in.

I was crying; he asked me what was wrong. He was friends with Amy's parents. He was their next-door neighbor.

"You wouldn't understand, I just want to go home."

The next day, the principal had a meeting with Amy and her parents. Someone else had reported what had happened. To this day, I still don't know who it was. He made the teacher change the seating plan. But Amy ended up getting my old desk and getting to sit by her friends.

At the end of the year, Amy won the peer mediation award, Melissa won the band award, and Camille won the academic award. I had a 97 percent average that year. I didn't win anything. I should have seen that one coming. The guidance counselor wouldn't look at me anymore; my homeroom teacher acted like nothing had ever happened. I left school that year and never looked back. Now we're in high school, and my ex-boyfriend is friends with Amy, Melissa, and Camille. I am alone, but I am victorious. I will never regret standing up for myself. I will never resent the consequences.

—AGE 16

We Can't Be Friends Anymore

Jenna and I have known each other since we were in preschool. We have gone to temple, school, camp, and for a while had Bat Mitzvah tutoring together. This past summer had been an interesting experience for both of us. Two summers ago, our second year at camp, we had to go to two different sessions. I had to go first session; she had to go second.

During that session, I met someone who would probably be my closest friend for the rest of my life. Her name was Amanda. Amanda and I were inseparable. The following year, when I found out we had to go different sessions, Amanda and I were both devastated; but then I found out Amanda would also be going to my session. I was the happiest person alive.

At the beginning of this past summer, I took a family cruise with my younger sister, mom, and dad. My sister, who is fourteen months younger than me, met some of the greatest friends in the world. They were from all over the country: one boy from Chicago, another from Texas, another from Georgia, another from Arkansas, and a girl from California. They were all in our age range, twelve to fourteen. We ran around the cruise ship with them all night. Once we got back from the cruise, my sister's and my mind had changed about people who live outside of our little, safe suburb.

At camp, I was so happy to see all my old friends. Plus, I got to see my best friend, Amanda. Things went great for a while. Then the trouble started. One Saturday, I wanted to head up to the camp's dining hall early to get a soda.

I kept on saying, "Jenna, I'll meet you up there. I just wanna get a soda quickly."

But she kept saying, "Julie, you have to wait for me." This went on for two or three minutes.

I finally said, "I'm going up to get a soda. I'll meet you up there." And I left. The main reason I left so quickly was I had to tell my sister about what just happened. For a few days Jenna and I argued, then finally we made up.

Then hell broke out again between the two of us. It was time to pick the activity we wanted for the second two weeks. The first time I did tennis and so did Jenna. My best friend Amanda and my other two friends, Daniella and Anna, and I decided to do music. We were so happy. We all loved to sing.

But the problem was I told Jenna I would do photography with her. I decided to lie to Jenna. The main reason I did this was because every time we were thinking of an idea I would say, "I wanna do drama," and she would say, "I wanna do drama, too." Then I would say, "Maybe I wanna do ceramics," and she would say, "I wanna do ceramics, too." This went on for about five activities.

I thought this was a good decision because at this time I had been getting very annoyed with her. Also, all my other friends agreed I should lie since I should have some time to be with people other than Jenna. Later, she asked what I had signed up for really. I told the truth and I said, "I'm sorry, I signed up for music." She started yelling at me again and we didn't speak for about a week. Just for the record, my performance went great. I stood up in front of the entire camp singing the first verse and chorus of "When You Believe" from *The Prince of Egypt*.

Now comes the last part of this epic story. It was the last Saturday of the session. My friends Elana, Anna, Daniella, Jenna, and I were sitting in one of the meeting halls at camp. Jenna had been sitting in the back, while the rest of us were messing around in the front doing our cartwheels and junk like that.

Jenna said something that we all interpreted as, "Julie, can you go give Amanda her water bottle?" I said no because I didn't know where she was at the moment.

Jenna suddenly said, "Julie, I was just asking you to give it to her!" I will use my exact words for this next part.

I said, "I'm not going to walk around the entire

fucking camp to give her something when we're both going to be seeing her at the same time!" She got mad and stomped out. I gave her the middle finger while she was walking out and I called her a bitch after she left.

Both of us were very mad. I was sick and tired of her and I wanted to dump her the next time I saw her. You need to know that I am 5' 3" and Jenna is 4' 10" and not the most fit person in the world. I could wrestle her to the ground and beat her up in a second if I wanted to. I found out later Daniella, Anna, and Elana had gotten annoyed with her, too, and had dumped her later that day.

You have to understand, I didn't turn them against her. The main things Jenna talked about were only meeting her grandparents once, about saying her sister was a pest, continually saying "guess what" before she told us anything, and saying "sissy," "horsy," "mommy," "daddy," and "doggie" all the time. You could stand it for about a minute, but soon you would think someone her age should be using more proper language and be a little more mature.

Jenna was liked by no one in our cabin. I had written my mom about all of these events and she told me we'd work it out at home, but for now, I should just have a great time.

A week before school started, our school had an orientation. My mom decided I should tell Jenna that we can't be as close as we were, but we can still be friends. I was planning to do that. But when Jenna and I started talking, I felt like it was old times. Then, when all my other friends came, I wanted her to get out of my sight.

Once school started, I was happy to see my friend I've known since kindergarten, Kathryn. Jenna, Kathryn, and I had the same gym class. Many times Jenna approached me and said, "I feel like you're ignoring me. Are you?" My reply was always, "Jenna, you have to understand I spent a month in a cabin with you and I haven't seen Kathryn for the entire summer." Her reply was always "Okay," but the question arose many times.

Then came Yom Kippur. My friend Jamie, from temple, asked a bunch of us over including me and Jenna. I was the only one who could make it because I would be going home with Jamie. Jenna couldn't make it, and I was very happy. But Jenna asked me how I was getting there and my reply was, "I'm going home with Jamie." She asked her parents about doing the same, and Jenna joined in. I was not very happy.

During gym that Tuesday, Jenna approached me and said, "Julie, you were so nice to me on Monday. Why are you ignoring me?" I couldn't stand it anymore. I finally said, "Jenna, I spent a month in a cabin with you and I didn't like it at all!" She, once again, pouted in her corner. To show her my aggressiveness, I stole the soccer ball from her and had an assist in soccer against her team.

That day I wrote a note to her saying we could not be friends anymore. She did not take it literally. She later wrote me a note that was mainly insults. Some things it said were: "Why is this problem only about you? I have feelings, too, you know." My thought was that I was the one who was having the problem with her in the first place. And another one was "You can't have people do stuff for you" (because I had another friend, Carrie, give her the note). "Don't you have guts? You needed to come to my face about it."

My reaction was, too much would come out. I would have said some pretty mean things to her. The day I got that letter I could not stand it anymore. The next day I went to her face and told her we couldn't be friends anymore. I was sick of dealing with this problem because it was putting too much stress on me and I couldn't focus on my schoolwork. I also felt like I couldn't be my own person with her always following me around.

Our gym teacher said we can come and talk to her when we want to, and I trust her more then my school counselor. Many times I have gone to talk to our gym teacher. Jenna continually has been wanting to sort out this problem, but you have to have two people to sort out the problem and both have to agree with it.

To this day, Jenna and I are still not friends. She still is giving both me *and* my sister evil glares. The glares to my sister are because my sister plays the same instruments as her. My sister is much better than Jenna. One day the orchestra teacher asked my sister to sit "first stand," which is an eighth grade stand and my sister is in seventh and Jenna is in eighth. Jenna should have been sitting first stand. Jenna was not very happy when that happened.

—AGE 14

Left Out, Left Behind

When you grow up in a society that tells you to be nice all the time, you not only fear saying you're upset—you probably don't even know how.

It's not just anger that girls struggle to express. It could be any unhappy feeling: jealousy, competition, feeling annoyed or offended, wanting to spend time with new friends, feeling like you've outgrown someone, and so on.

When something is hard to say, a lot of girls get quiet. It happens all of a sudden, like a blackout. One minute there's light, and everything's cool; the next it's pitch black and it's undeniable something's changed. You don't know where to go or what to do.

Girls get quiet because they're afraid to say what they really think. In *Odd Girl Out,* I asked girls why they didn't say how they were feeling directly. They replied, "I'm afraid to say something I don't mean," or "I'm afraid she won't be my friend anymore." An overwhelming number of girls believed direct conflict would cause people to abandon or hate them.

That's why when you go up to your friend and ask her if she's mad, the answer is usually no. Or she says she's not really ignoring you or being weird, or whatever it is you suspect she's doing. She is upset, but she's afraid of what will happen if she tells you, so she leaves you in this strange no-man's-land, neither here nor there. She makes you feel crazy. You're sure you know what's going on, but she's telling you otherwise. You want to believe her, but you can't shake the sinking feeling in your stomach that something is really, really wrong.

When girls outgrow each other, it usually happens like this: You used to be so close, and all of a sudden she's not there anymore. She's with other people at lunch, on the weekend, on the playground. She's distracted, looking over at others while she's hanging with you. The new girls are probably more popular. You ask your friend what's up and she says, "Nothing!" or "I'm just getting to know some other people." And: "I'm *not* mad."

First of all, you're not crazy. I promise. Believe what you see.

Most girls think it's their fault. You must have done something to make her abandon you like this.

You didn't.

Clearly, you think, you're a total loser: not cool enough, not pretty enough, not enough of anything.

You aren't.

Did you ever hear of the Sirens in Greek mythology? They were three girls beached on a tiny island, and they had incredible singing voices. In fact, they sang so sweetly that anyone who sailed by, minding their own business, was entranced.

People couldn't help themselves. They had to get closer to those voices, and they forgot everything: their missions, their values, their own names. Once they reached the Sirens, the ladies killed them. Even after the Sirens got a reputation for seduction and murder, people still sailed hypnotically toward their voices. They couldn't think about anything else, and they wanted nothing more.

Popularity is like one of the Sirens. Your friend who's slipping away from you is in its clutches. She's spellbound by popularity, and she'll do anything to get and stay with the in crowd or person.

It's not that she doesn't like you. In all likelihood, her feelings for you haven't changed. When you hang out together on your own, it's probably just like old times. But when she gets around Her, or Them, she's different.

That's not about you. It's about her. This situation happens all the time to many different kinds of girls, and it's one of the most painful social experiences you can have.

It's certainly possible that you did do something to cause this rift, and in that case you should try to figure out what. I'm not telling you to pretend nothing is wrong. What I'm saying is there's a difference between feeling bad and blaming yourself, and feeling bad because you've been hurt by someone.

Is your friend a bully because she's acting this way? Not unless she's dissing you openly or behind your back with her new pals. She probably wants to find a way to be your friend and Their friend. Or she might be moving on.

The question is: Are you willing to accept the way she's treating you? Right now, the friendship is probably happening on her terms. In other words, your friend says when you'll hang out. She says when you won't. She's nice to you when she wants to be. She controls the rules of the relationship.

Now you have to decide if you want to give her that control.

Before you act, here are some things to keep in mind: People are allowed to make new friends. BFF doesn't mean only-friendship-I-have-no-one-else-allowed. Just because your friend wants to hang out with other people doesn't mean she's leaving you behind. But it doesn't give you automatic access to all her new friends either.

If you can accept that there will be other people in her life besides you, you can play an active role in finding a way to be friends that will make both of you feel good. No matter how bad you feel, don't forget that she's probably struggling, too. If you don't admit to that, and accept that you may have to compromise, too, you might not save your friendship.

I have two very close girlfriends I met in college. Maggie is my roommate in Brooklyn and Jenny lives down the street. Years ago, after some awkward situations, we realized that sometimes we liked "alone time" in pairs. We agreed that there was pleasure in being one-on-one and having a unique connection to someone. Sometimes it made me uncomfortable, for sure, but we agreed that anyone who felt hurt or took it personally was reading too much into it. If we needed to, we talked about our feelings of exclusion. Eventually, we all got used to the arrangement, and now it feels normal, even easy.

Perhaps you need to make a similar arrangement with your friends. A lot of girls judge the strength of their friendships by how often they hang out, and that's a mistake. If your friend decides to spend time with someone else, it doesn't mean she doesn't like you as much, or that she's talking about you behind your back.

The more you freak out about it, the more you cling to someone, the more turned off your friend gets. And if it scares you that your friend isn't spending time with you the way she used to, the answer is to find another friend to fill some of those empty spaces—and to work on easing the insecurity you feel.

You might try asking your friend if she prefers to

spend time alone with her new friends, and if that's true, ask if you could arrange for your own alone time together. Maybe you could have a standing date when you hang out or talk, like Maggie and Jenny do. They have dinner together every Monday night.

If you need to have a serious talk, both of you must commit to asking yourselves and each other some hard questions. On a piece of paper, try writing thoughtful answers to the following:

- What is she doing that is making me feel sad, hurt, angry, annoyed, or [fill in the blank]?

- What do I want her to do differently?

- What can I do for myself to make this change in our friendship easier?

- What am I doing that is making her feel sad, hurt, angry, annoyed, or [fill in the blank]?

- What could I do differently to make our friendship better?

- What can I do for her that would make this change in our friendship easier?

Both of you have to answer every single question, even if you think you can't possibly come up with the answer. You may look at the questions and sigh and feel angry and want to crumple up the paper and feed it to your dog, but when you're done feeling frustrated, sit down again and think about it.

When you're ready, talk together about your answers. If you find your talk dissolving into a fight, check out page 148 for some tips on better listening. Even if your friend isn't willing to answer the questions, use your answers to express your feelings to her, in a letter or in person.

Let's say things aren't going quite so smoothly. Your friendship may not be like old times, even when you're one-on-one. Maybe your friend ignores you when her new posse or friend is around, puts you down, or tells them your secrets. Let's say you try improving the situation using suggestions from earlier in this section, but nothing changes. Then you've got an entirely different situation on your hands, and you should consider other options.

One of the distinctive characteristics of female aggression is how often it shows up in close relationships. As a result, many girls wind up in abusive friendships. They put up with terrible treatment for months, even years. They often justify staying in the friendship by telling themselves that there are still good times, or that the friend says she's sorry or really can't help it.

There is no acceptable reason why you should ever be mistreated by a friend; it's nothing short of bullying. It's especially serious when the person doing it to you is your friend. When you're close with someone, they have a lot of power over you: They can influence your feelings about yourself, and your sense of inner peace and comfort. When someone you're close to degrades you repeatedly, or makes you feel bad about yourself, it's no longer friendship.

When you allow your "friend" to do this to you, consider the messages you're sending to her, and to the world, about yourself.

a. You deserve to be loved on someone else's terms, or according to someone else's rules.

b. You don't deserve to be liked all the time, or in a consistent way.

Is this what you think about yourself? Is this the person you want to be? Many girls grow up thinking this is a friendship, but ask yourself: Would you treat someone this way? So why are you putting up with it? Are you afraid of making other friends? Okay, almost everyone is. Crossing the lunchroom to sit at a new table seems to rank up there with jumping out of an airplane in a parachute made out of Kleenex. Trust me on this: It's not nearly as bad as you think.

What it comes down to is believing in yourself. Loving yourself. Thinking that, hey, I am a really good friend. I'm fun, loving, trustworthy, and loyal. If you don't think these things about yourself, it's hard to pick someone who will do the same. Everyone likes to say that the mean girls have low self-esteem—that they're jealous, or otherwise in a bad place in life. But what about you? If you're putting up with the way these mean girls treat you, what does that say about the way you feel about yourself? If you are worried that you do not value yourself enough, or if you need help getting out of a bad situation, please see page 178.

You may not be ready now, tomorrow, or even in a month. But when you are, remember: You have the right to explain to your friend exactly what you don't like about the ways she's treating you. You have the right to respectfully but firmly ask her to stop. And if she doesn't, you have the right to stop speaking to her and being her friend.

Setting Boundaries: Changing or Ending a Friendship

What if you're the one outgrowing your friend? It's probably a really exciting time for you. You've met some cool new people, and maybe you feel like they understand you, or bring something out in you, that no one ever has. You're having that thrilling rush of falling into friendship, and you couldn't be happier— except for the fact that your old friend is coming up to you and constantly harassing you to hang out, or asking why you're ignoring her, and you're sick of her following you around.

What are you supposed to do? Well, it depends. I don't envy your situation. You have a right to make other friends. Wanting to and doing it doesn't automatically make you a bully. The question is how you're going to make the transition.

First, ask yourself: Do you want to stay friends with her? I mean, really stay friends with her? That means a friendship on terms you both agree to: not just in private or when your new friends aren't around; not just when it's good for you, but a friendship that acknowledges what you both want.

If you're ready to do that, talk to your friend honestly about what's really going on. As I mentioned earlier, many girls in your shoes deny what's happening to their friends. They assure them that everything's the same. This isn't fair to either of you: to her because you're lying, and she's going to feel crazy because she knows something is different, and to you because you're lying, and you'll feel increasingly as though you have done something very wrong. You will quickly start to resent her because she will get in your way, annoy you, and make you feel bad about yourself.

The only alternative is honesty, and though it won't be easy at first, the long-term payoff is well worth it. I suggest you try saying something like the following.

"I love being friends, and I'm not trying to drop you. But I've met some new people that I am really into, and I want some alone time with them. I still want to hang out with you, and I'm not mad at you. Just because I spend time with other people doesn't mean we aren't still really close. No one else can have what we share because it's ours. What can I do to make this easier for you?"

Listen carefully to what she says. As an alternative, try suggesting you both answer the questions on page 53. Sit down together and talk about your answers. Try to hammer out a compromise that will allow you to stay friends on healthier terms. If you can, ask your guidance counselor to help you through the conversation.

What if your new friends have made you realize you've outgrown your old friend? What if you want to move on completely? You are entitled to end a friendship with someone, but again, it's all about how you do it. You'll have to accept certain realities that may make you very uncomfortable.

First, you will not be able to avoid hurting your friend, no matter how much you pretend it's not happening. She will feel sad, even devastated, about losing you.

Second, you have to tell her directly what is going on. You can't deny it. The more you withhold, the more you hurt her.

Third, don't, under any circumstances, send her mixed messages. What does that mean? If you're going to stop being friends with her, make the decision and stick to it. If you see her at some point and start acting like you're friends—like at a family function or church or anywhere you have no one else to hang out with—you are confusing and hurting her. You're making it hard for her to move on and accept the decision you've made.

That doesn't mean you should ignore her when you see her. It's fine to ask how she's doing and make small talk. But if you start laughing about inside jokes, telling secrets, and acting close, you're actually being mean, not nice. You ended the friendship, and you have every right to do that, but it's your responsibility to make and stick to boundaries.

What are boundaries? They're invisible lines you draw and don't cross. In a romantic relationship, boundaries set limits on any number of things, such as how far you want to go sexually, and when. Girls have trouble with boundaries in friendships because girls are raised to be nice to everyone and be everyone's friend. But that's hardly fair. Everyone has the right to set limits. No one can be everything to everyone.

Fourth, some people—especially your friend's mom—may call you mean, a bitch, or a bully for ending the friendship. We still live in a world that expects girls to be friends with everyone, and you may face a backlash. But as long as you stick to these boundaries, you are doing nothing wrong.

If you end the friendship by being mean to your old friend—talking about her behind her back with your new friends, revealing her secrets, pointing or whispering or laughing at her while she's around, getting the other girls to ignore or be mean to her—you are indeed bullying her. There is no excuse for turning other people against her, no matter how frustrated you may feel. Talk to a parent or counselor about her if you need to, not her peers. You may think she won't find out when you talk about her behind her back, but how do you know your new friends won't try to "help you out" by letting her know just what you think?

She Copied Me

"Ewwww, look at her. She's got such frizzy, red hair. Hee hee!" That's what my friends and I would always say about Mara. Well, at least that's what we thought. Every day of fourth grade she would follow us, mimic us, copy us, and try too hard in front of us.

It was at the end of fourth grade when it happened. All my friends and I got together and talked about why we didn't like Mara. We all tried to "hide" from her, but it kept getting worse. Don't think that it was just little things. They were huge things that really made us mad. Until one day, I had enough! She was buying the same exact clothes as me. She cut and styled her hair like me! I couldn't stand it! My friends talked to her, and the teacher, but after that she kept "clinging" to us even more. So one day I decided to go to the guidance counselor. We talked and talked, and finally brought Mara in with just two of us. I could tell that she was really getting sad.

At the end of the guidance, Mara just looked at me and said, "Why?" I told her that me and my friends had tried so many times to be her friend (which we had), but it just didn't work out. If trying to be her friend was that hard, I couldn't imagine being her friend.

So, the next year in fifth grade, Mara stopped acting like us and talking to us. At first we were all really happy, but then realized that we wanted someone mimicking us and trying too hard. But there was nothing we could do about it.

In conclusion, I give advice to those out there who have someone copying you: just wait, they could become your friend. I obviously made the wrong choice. And to those of you who are the ones trying too hard, don't. If the people don't like you for who you are, then don't bother being their friend. You are special in your own way.

—AGE 12

Just to Make You Happy

This must be a dream because you are here, in front of me. You are talking, talking so sweet and gentle; but whom are you talking to? To me? Really? Wow! Not many people talk to me, really. At least, not many people like you. You're perfect, you see, and I am full of flaws. You are everything a girl could dream of, and I am just one of those girls. Yet, you're talking to *me*; but why? I just don't understand. You have never talked to me before. You won't hear me complaining. I am lost in your deep, brown eyes. Everything is so real, but how can it be?

I know you must be telling me something simple, like, I am in your way. Strangely, I hear no words coming from your mouth. I'm staring, but I can't help it. We've made eye contact and I want to devote my life to not breaking it. I still can't believe it! You've never given me so much as a passing glance and now you are actually saying words to me. No, not words, sentences! I listen to your voice that flows like honey, but it seems you are speaking a foreign language.

What are you saying? I come back to reality just in time to hear you say, "...over." Excuse me? What did you say? Why are you giving me that look? Oh, please don't, it breaks my heart. You unhappily repeat what you said. You want *me* to move over so you can sit by your friends. Of course! I would do anything for you. Just to make you happy.

—AGE 13

Small Town Clique

My name is Jane. I'm fourteen and live in a culturally and racially mixed town close to New York. I have two older sisters and one younger brother, and we all live together in a traditional family setting. I'm very athletic — people would say "tomboyish." I roller blade, long board, surf, swim, and play soccer and basketball.

I attended a relatively small grammar school and always had plenty of friends, both boys and girls. I was especially close to Jessica, who I considered my best friend. She was the "It" girl. In third grade I was diagnosed with a learning disability, dyslexia. This didn't affect me socially until sixth grade.

I was the only sixth grader who had to go to a special teacher and classroom once a day for remedial help. Boys started to pass negative comments about me leaving the class to go for "special help." It was humiliating, to say the least. I never received any different treatment from the girls, or at least I didn't notice it.

For seventh and eighth grade we have to go to a junior high school, and so do three other grammar schools in our town. I took to junior high pretty well. I met a lot of new girls and was beginning to enjoy myself. I slowly noticed my close "It" girlfriends were calling less and less.

In school, people started to notice that I was in a resource room for three classes and the embarrassment was worse than before. I have been called "sped" (special ed.), my class has been referred to as the retard class, and remarks have been made about my books being different from other kids'.

Eventually, I got close to and felt comfortable with one girl, Lily, who also was being left out of her original group. I thought everything was going to be okay until I returned from my Easter vacation. I found that even Lily had dropped me when she was let back into the "It" group.

I was very hurt, sad, and confused. I did a lot of crying that year.

My mom made me and my sisters watch the *Oprah* show on aggressive girls. After the show I cried and told my mom, "It would be nice just to be included."

I'm doing better in eighth grade, not socially but emotionally. I try not to let it bother me as much and I have two very good friends, Alexis and Maddy, who live down the Jersey Shore. I keep in contact with them as much as possible. They help me deal with everything, but I find it funny, because they've experienced it, too. I guess "mean girls" are everywhere. It seems to happen to everyone at least once.

I believe I was cut out of the popular girl group because of my learning disability. I think about it a lot and realize there's nothing that can be done to change it. I've asked to be taken out of the resource program but at the same time I know I need the help and the social damage has been done.

I know that in time my life will change and move forward, but I'm not so sure theirs will.

—AGE 14

Popularity and Gossip

I've always known I wasn't the most popular person. In fact, to me, being popular is something I probably could never be. I'm just not "popular" material. I bet that you've always wanted to know the quiet girl's point of view, so here it is....

Popularity — To me, popularity means that you have a lot of friends and have to look decent. Do I envy popular people? Of course. It doesn't bother me that much anymore, though. Are popular people mean? Some are, some aren't. It depends on what school you're in, and who the person is. I've seen both nice and mean people. The nice populars tend to be sympathy nice. They have that worried sound in their voice, or throw a random comment at you. I hate it when they throw random comments at you. I suppose they are only trying to be nice to others.

The mean populars tend to be nice to you, then turn around and start talking about you. They don't seem to notice that the person can see or hear them.

It's especially annoying when people turn to someone, whisper in their ear, and stare at you while doing so. Then, out of the "kindness of their heart," the person receiving info looks at you and says something like, "You don't want to know what she's saying." *That* really annoys me.

Gossip — Gossip is easily spread around, especially in my school because it is small. You have to be careful what you tell, and whom you tell. I suggest not telling any deep dark secrets to your buddies, because even if you don't want to believe it, it's going to spread across the school. In many cases, one fact is somehow twisted into this forty-minute story on something that was a simple one sentence thing. So try not to tell too many people about your problems, 'cause the next thing you know, everyone's going to be staring at you and you will be knocking on the counselor's door. The reason for this is that people need something to talk about, to use against you, to brag about, to tell on you, so forth and so on.

About Me — In my view, I am the quiet girl sitting next to you. I am a very shy person, so I usually don't have a lot of friends. It's just my nature; I can't help it. I mean sure, I want to have a lot of friends, be popular and funny, gossip and have fun (which I have anyway). But it's hard for me, so tough luck. Most of my friends are popular.

My feelings are easily hurt, though I often don't show it. I'm not depressed or anything, just easily offended. Though many people don't seem to understand it, I know what they say about me, I know when they whisper about me. I mean, when you whisper in someone's ear, and both of them are staring at you, it is a little obvious, you know.

I know who thinks what of me. I've got connections. I've always been nice to people, even the ones that openly express their hate for me. I've done a variety of things from picking up books to helping with homework, going to a teacher and buying candy for someone else, giving them some of my food, and so on. Some people just don't understand me. That doesn't bother me. It doesn't bother me that people talk about me, or that I'm not popular, or that I'm misunderstood. It just bothers me that some people don't recognize what I do for them, even though they treat me like dirt.

—AGE 13

Stone by Stone

You are very dear to my heart.
I felt like I could tell you anything
Right from the start.
We talked about everything together,
From our "deepest darkest secrets"
To crying on each other's shoulders because of
    something our parents said.
You were always there for me,
And I was always there for you.
When people said your name,
They said mine, too.
We were inseparable.

Until one day,
You said you liked him,
But I liked him, too,
Were we to let a silly little boy come between us?
All of our memories,
All of our secrets shared,
Gone?

Because of a boy?
I guess so,
I guess that's how things go when you're a crazy
	teenage girl.

But why?
The way his hair falls in front of his face?
That drives me crazy, too.
Is it the way when his hand brushes yours, you tingle
	all over?
Yup, I love that, too.
Or is it the way he always seems to notice just you, in
	a crowd of people?
That's the best feeling, isn't it?
I know exactly how he makes you feel.
Trust me, I feel the same way.

This doesn't mean he has to come between our
	endless nights
Of talking.
The endless tears shed from our eyes, or
The nonreplaceable friendship that we have built,
Step by step,
Stone by stone.
It takes more than a boy to crumble the wall we've
	built.
It is too strong,
Too intense,
To fall because of a boy.

—AGE 15

Let Me Create Myself

I walked into school
And she smiled.
I thought to myself
Who could be this child?

She is not like the others
All looking down
Yes, she is very different
Not wearing a frown.

I stand there listening
So silently
For if I say the wrong thing
They will surely ignore me.

I am unhappy with myself
Trying so hard to fit in
I try to look like them
But I can never win.

She smiles happily
At me once again

She makes me feel
As though we're friends.

On the same team I never talked
To her when we played tennis.
The other girls thought of her
As unpopular and a menace.

I finally decided
No more people creating me
Let me create myself
The way I want to be.

I walked up to her
And said let's be friends
She nodded and I knew
This friendship would never end.

The sun is now shining
The clouds are all gone
This friendship is so special
That I have fell upon.

I am thankful for her teaching me
How to be myself and care
But what I am most thankful for
Is the *true* friendship that we share.

—AGE 15

You'll Be Missed . . .

Some people come into our lives and quickly go.
Some people stay for a while, and give us a
deeper understanding of what is truly important in
this life. They touch our souls. We gain strength
from the footprints they have left on our hearts,
and we will never EVER be the same.

— Author Unknown

Bike riding, gymnastics classes, endless games of pretend . . . my best friend and I did it all; we were inseparable. Growing up across the street from each other made it easy for us to play every day after school, on the weekends, and throughout the summer.

As young and carefree kids we would spend our afternoons playing with Barbies and setting up lemonade stands. As time went on, we replaced dolls with basketballs and tennis rackets. We discussed our dreams of making it to the Olympics and practiced against any neighbor boys willing. Of course this phase, along with the numerous others, soon came to an end.

We approached middle school, and all of a sudden, grades, *boys,* and name-brand clothes became way too big of a deal. We would still see each other daily, but we spent our time sitting in her room or mine talking for endless hours. She was always there for me; she was without a doubt my best friend.

One day something that had merely been small talk for months became a reality . . . she was moving. Her family was simply relocating to a different area of the same city, but to me it seemed as if she was moving to a different country. She would not be at next year's block party, or there to sled down our huge hill after the winter's first snowfall.

We planned on spending every second before her move together, but we were both in for a surprise when one day, out of the blue, we got into a huge fight. I still don't understand what our argument was about, and I don't remember exactly what was said, but I will never forget how much I was hurt as my best friend—since I was born, basically—said she feels uncomfortable around me and never wants to see me again.

Being only in seventh grade I was hurt, confused, and alone. When I needed my friend the most, needed the advice and support, she was no longer there. Once she moved we talked briefly online, but within a few months we looked at each other as strangers and the following year we did not speak more than ten words to each other.

When I found out she had decided to go to the same high school I was going to attend, I wondered if our friendship would resume or if we would remain distant. One summer day before our freshman year, I received a letter from my old friend. It came as a surprise as I read her words apologizing and telling me how she had realized how much I used to be a part of her life. She wanted our friendship back if at all possible.

Holding back confusion, hurt feelings, and grudges, I agreed that I, too, needed her in my life again. It was really awkward at first; I even felt uncomfortable hanging around her because of our past, and I knew she felt the same way.

At high school we quickly became a part of two close but different cliques. The two groups still did a lot together and as time passed we worked out our differences and once again became close. We will never again be the same two girls who spent hours in the woods building forts or sleeping outdoors in tents, but at least we had each other to share laughs and to fall back on for support.

My friend is currently going through a rough time. One of her many obstacles has been the divorce of her parents. Because our families were such good friends, it killed me to see hers fall apart.

As a result, she is now moving with her mom, stepfather, and sisters — 402 miles and five hours and forty minutes from our little road in Missouri. I now realize how lucky we had it when she was only moving out of the neighborhood.

My friend is smart, athletic, well liked, and incredibly talented; she is always fun to be around! I have total confidence that she will thrive in her new environment and daily become closer to the numerous dreams she has set for herself. I am just sad to lose her.

I write this story so others can realize the importance of their friends. I had to lose mine to understand how much it meant to have a *best friend*. Don't take anything or anyone for granted. Let your friends know what they mean to you and that you'll always be there for them.

Thanks to the Internet, I hope my friend and I will be able to stay in contact. I only hope she knows how thankful I am to have had her as a friend. I will always be here for her!

—AGE 16

"A NEVER-ENDING NIGHTMARE"

When Friends Turn On You

If you find yourself at school one day and your friends are ignoring you, and no one will tell you why, and even when you find out why and try to apologize no one seems to care, what can you do?

A lot of times, not much. When girls get angry like that—and you will know in your gut if they are that angry—they are hard to stop. They have probably been quietly angry for a long time, and now that it's out in the open, they're going to have a lot to say.

The writers in this section explore the grief, fear, and fury that define the moment when your friends turn on you. Next to food, water, and for some girls, a full-length mirror, friends are the most important part of a girl's existence. It's not uncommon for girls to say things like, "My friends are my life." When your friends are suddenly gone, a lot of girls say their lives are over. I don't blame them.

Girlfriends help you survive parents, school, guys, and everything in between. When you're feeling fat and ugly, your friends say you look fine. When you're freaking out about grades, your friends tell you how smart you are.

When your friends are gone, everything about your life looms larger. Things that you could deal with are suddenly scary. Things that were hard before now seem impossible. Some of the writers in this section describe going through a truly traumatic experience that led to depression and eating disorders. Others take their pain as a sign that girls are not to be trusted, ever.

In spite of their sadness, many writers looking back tell us how pain taught them important life lessons. One writes, "I wouldn't take back anything I went through because I have gained so much through my struggle. I've gained so much more understanding for people. No longer do I judge or label. I am open to everything and everyone; I want to help people who are experiencing what I am, and most importantly I want everyone to know that no matter how bad things seem, they do get better...I got better."

For those who can't yet look back, I include some advice on how to deal, now and afterward. Your silver lining is out there.

The Missing Friend

Who's that girl standing apart from me
Why she's my friend or she used to be
I told her everything I know, who I like and so
    and so
And then one day, right out of the blue
She no longer liked me, she gave me no clue
Why have you left me, have I done something wrong
I remember our friendship like it were a song
Even though now all she does is stare
I can't help but wonder
Does she remember all the memories we share

—AGE 11

I Was in a Never-Ending Nightmare

There's always that one person in every school. The person who gets made fun of and judged when no one really knows much about them. The feelings this person has from the taunting and teasing are more than anyone could ever imagine going through. The pain classmates can cause these days is unbelievable. At my school, that student was me.

Last summer (the summer between seventh and eighth grade), my closest girlfriends seemed to drop me overnight. I would go to the beach and I would see the girls who had been my best friends all through seventh grade, but now they were hanging out with another clique from another school. Every time I went to the beach and walked past this clique of girls, they would call me a whore and just ramble on about how gross I was. The girls who used to be my best friends would just sit there and say nothing. There had been so many times when I was there for them, but now they wouldn't stand up for me. They let these popular girls insult me, and they just sat there silently. Later, they admitted to the school social worker that they weren't courageous enough to go against the new clique. I guess they just desperately wanted to be part of this popular group.

On the first day of school I thought that this year — eighth grade — would be the turning over of a new leaf. I wished that I'd be popular just like last year. I hoped for a new and better reputation. People had heard some things about what I had done with boys over the summer, and not all of them were true. But everyone believed all of the rumors. This changed everything. Kids would come up to me and call me a whore to my face as well as try to trip me in the halls. My classmates would also make obscene, disgusting gestures about sexual behaviors that they believed I'd done. They would talk about me constantly, whispering about the rumors they had heard, staring at me, and laughing right when they were doing it. My few friends and I were very confused about why people kept bothering me. I decided just to ignore it all and see what happened.

As things got worse, I realized I could not ignore it, and so I decided to talk with the school social worker about what was going on. She understood me very well and encouraged me to go with my first plan, which was to ignore it. I tried again to ignore the teasing and the gossip and the harassment, but things got out of hand. Kids would write horrible things on desks about me and write notes about me and put them in front of my locker purposely so I could see what they had written about me. For example, they'd write that I was a dirty whore. One girl who used to be a good friend of mine said she couldn't hang out with me anymore because I'd "made big mistakes." I thought to myself, "But everybody makes mistakes!" Why couldn't my friends just stick by me and support me through my hard times? I'd made a few mistakes with boys, but so had some other seventh and eighth grade girls, and the things the kids were saying about me were exaggerated and cruel. It was like they needed a scapegoat, and so they chose me.

Soon my classmates started to tease me about other things that weren't to be made fun of. When I was in seventh grade, I started to become depressed, and most of my friends knew I had clinical depression. I was very open about it because that's what I was taught to do in my family. Most of my friends knew that over the summer (before eighth grade), I had started taking an antidepressant, and my friends and classmates had at first been very supportive and sympathetic about it all. But now, everyone was acting like I was crazy, when the truth was that I had a biochemical illness that I had no control over. When kids saw me in the hall, they would make cruel gestures, pretending to slit their wrists. Some girls started calling me "psycho" and they told other girls who were being nice to me that I would mess them up and make them crazy, too. I tried to tell my classmates that depression was definitely not something to make fun of. It's an illness, just like any other illness. I told them that you don't see people making fun of someone who has cancer or diabetes, do you? Depression is just like cancer: It's an illness, and it isn't funny.

I didn't understand why any of this was taking place. Why was I the target here? I didn't do anything to get kids upset with me. Why was everyone being so harsh? I was so confused about why they seemed so driven to tear me apart.

All of my girlfriends began to drop me. They wouldn't sit next to me at lunch and wouldn't call me or write me notes and e-mails. If I sat down at the same table as them, they would gather their things and leave. These were girls who used to be my best friends! All of a sudden the phone calls at home were never for me. My Friday nights and weekends turned into staying home, watching television with my parents, and cleaning my room. I would try calling my friends, but they'd say they were busy. Things got lonely and I felt hopeless. It got to the point where I couldn't go through the halls without a laugh, a cough disguising a mean name, a whisper, a trip, a gesture, or a shout. My classmates would threaten me and would throw volleyballs at me at recess, and the playground supervisors wouldn't do a thing.

At recess or during class, I would go to the bathroom and cry in the stall for twenty minutes or so.

Everything felt closed in and lonely. It was like I was in a never-ending nightmare. I was buried in a cold black hole where no one cared or understood.

Things got so intense that I ended up running to the school social worker sobbing almost every period, every day. I went to the principal and assistant principal as well. They decided to talk to some kids to try to stop the bullying. But nothing seemed to work. Kids would still bother me as well as bully and tease me. And the girls who used to be my friends kept ignoring me and excluding me.

By the middle of November, things became so unbearable at school that I begged my parents to let me stay home from school. I was too depressed to go to school. My parents had tried for almost three months to work with the principal and the social worker, but things were not improving. So my parents finally decided to take drastic measures by taking me out of school. My parents totally supported me on this just as they had through all of it. They decided to homeschool me for the rest of eighth grade. Homeschooling seemed to be the healthiest option for me.

When all this happened to me, I was angry because I didn't think that I should be the one missing my education. I thought the kids who teased and verbally bullied me should be the ones suspended and missing their education. But none of the kids were suspended, and the school I had attended since kindergarten was no longer an environment that I felt safe in. What I went through isn't acceptable and shouldn't be allowed.

At first I thought that by leaving my school, I was letting my classmates win. But as I thought more about the situation, I realized that I was the one who won. I had left an unacceptable situation and moved on with my life and put all of this behind me. I decided I was not going to let my life be defined by this group of kids and this school. It has taken me several months to build self-esteem and to realize that leaving the school was a sign of strength, not a sign of weakness.

Because of this experience I have learned many things. I've always known that bullying was bad. But now that I've been a victim of it, I totally agree that emotional as well as physical bullying is wrong. Bullying can create scars that last a long time. What someone is or what someone isn't is nothing to make fun of. And I believe that every kid in America needs to learn that.

I also learned that being popular isn't everything. Sometimes you can learn a lot more meaningful lesson by going solo. Another thing I learned is that if something is wrong or you are being teased at school or anywhere else, you should always tell an adult so they can help.

—AGE 14

Who My Friends Really Were

The group of girls I hung out with had a weird way of doing things. It was almost like there were rules you had to follow, unwritten rules, and if you broke one you would be punished. For as long as I could remember, I followed these rules; I followed them to the best of my ability, with extra effort, hoping that I would somehow be included more than I was. I had to be friends with all of them; doing something separate was breaking a rule and in turn left me punished. I wouldn't be talked to for days nor would I be called on weekends. Notes would be passed and even given to me explaining how angry they were. Everything got twisted and the truth never made it out. Everyone was turned against me before I even had a chance to tell my side of the story.

It's funny though, how you go along with it when it isn't you or when it doesn't directly affect you. When I was the one accepted and ignoring another, never did I once care how that person felt, never did I once relate the pain I would feel to theirs. It simply didn't matter to me; I was perfectly happy and content with the fact that it wasn't me this time.

November of 2001 is when I started to have feelings of withdrawal. I wanted to be alone all the time. At first I didn't understand it, nor did I connect my ongoing weight loss to it. I figured it was just a phase I was going through. As for the weight... I was a teenage girl, what girl wouldn't like to lose a couple pounds? Well, the couple pounds turned into six, then six turned into twelve, and then it wouldn't stop. I felt sad all the time and there would be days when I wouldn't want to stop crying. I went through this alone for three months, telling no one what I felt, and denying anything was wrong with me. My social life was at zero. What once was a bubbly girl had turned into a girl who attended only what was required. I remember days that I would go to school, and I wouldn't even talk. No one seemed to notice or care.

It wasn't until February that I figured out there was a cause for what I was feeling. I was diagnosed with clinical depression. What scary words! I didn't understand how I, someone that used to be so happy, could have something so scary. Depression isn't something that you cause, and it is definitely not your fault. Depression is caused by a chemical imbalance in your brain. Everyone experiences some type of depression throughout their life, but most people can deal with it and get out of it. For me, depression had taken over my life.

Food had lost its taste, and I in turn had lost my ambition to eat. My trim athletic 117 pounds had turned into eighty-seven pounds. None of my clothes fit and you could see every bone in my body. I hated the way I looked; it was never a matter of body image or a way for me to gain attention. I wanted so badly to have my old life back.

My friends noticed my dramatic change but didn't seem to care. It was something that we didn't talk about; it was something they talked about behind my back. They knew something was wrong but didn't know how to approach it. I was labeled anorexic, and I left it that way. I thought it would be easier to be called "Ana" a couple times than to try to explain to them what I was actually feeling. This went on for a good six months.

I don't know why in those six months I expected my friends to support me; maybe it was because that was what real friends were supposed to do. Maybe they didn't support me because they were never real friends. I know I was never their first choice; I was rather a last resort person, a person they would call when no one else was around to do anything. However, even these calls had stopped. All the pain I had felt before from not being included some of the time had been turned into constant pain from not ever being included. I never knew anything different than what I had; they were my world, and they were "my friends." I couldn't possibly imagine my life without them. When they stopped talking and calling me, it was like my world had ended.

These months allowed me to experience what it was like to be left out all the time; I realized how unfair and cruel everything was. However, with these realizations, I would still hide my problem, and I still wanted more than ever to be a part of the group again. I thought I was good at covering these things up, too. I'd wear big clothes to hide my body and I'd try and smile when people occasionally said hi. I felt so alone inside. There were times when I didn't want to be here anymore; there were times when I didn't want even to give the effort of getting up in the morning. Everything required energy, something I didn't have, and something I couldn't have at such a low body weight.

I think my "friends" really realized how bad it was when we started swimming in gym class. I couldn't even swim a lap without getting tired. I was freezing and nothing I did could make me warm. The thinness of my body was only intensified by my being in a swimsuit. I only swam one time; I couldn't take it emotionally or physically. I would always hear the whispers and the cruel things people would say about me. My body couldn't take me burning off the calories I so desperately needed.

The library became first block class instead of P.E.; from that day forward I was forced to sit by myself in the library hoping *that* would somehow put weight back on my body. What people didn't realize was that this only worsened my depression; I was now totally separated from everyone and everything.

I don't know how I got through the school year but I did. Things started to get better for me. I saw a therapist for my emotional problems and a nutritionist for the physical problems. It seemed once I was okay and stopped hiding the problem, the weight started to come back. I realized so many things — when you go through something so tough you tend to realize things. I realized when my friends wouldn't help me through, what fake friendships I actually had. I realized the importance of family and how no matter what, they will always love you and be there for you. One thing I didn't realize or deal with yet was letting go of these friendships I'd had for so long, even if they were fake.

It was the Fourth of July when I finally couldn't deal with the "friendships" anymore. I had sprained my ankle earlier in the day and was on crutches. The group had planned to go watch the fireworks together. I was excited because I was finally invited to something again; after so long they had called me and asked me if I wanted to come along. I began to think this was finally all over; because I was getting better I would be back in the swing of things soon... I had no idea how wrong I was. That evening the girls decided to walk to the fireworks, knowing that I couldn't walk and knowing that this would mean I couldn't go along. Something that would usually cause tears, instead caused a feeling of freedom. I looked at my still-emaciated body in the mirror and told myself it was my turn — my turn to feel special, my turn to feel wanted, and my turn to do it all by myself, without the girls who had brought me down so much.

The rest of the summer I built friendships with kids I knew from church, kids I worked with, and whoever else I could. People I wouldn't ever think of talking to before had become my best friends. Once I stepped out of my carbon-copy image I was more accepting of everyone else. It seemed great. However, summer had ended and I had to go back to school. I had to go back to seeing those girls every day.

I didn't want to have to deal with this anymore, I didn't want to have to deal with them, and most of all I didn't want to have to deal with the pain. I chose to go to a new school, not because I was running away but because I wanted a place where I could just start over, where I could finally just be accepted for who I really was.

I wouldn't take back anything I went through because I have gained so much through my struggle. I've gained so much more understanding for people. No longer do I judge or label. I am open to everything and everyone; I want to help people who are experiencing what I am, and most importantly I want everyone to know that no matter how bad things seem, they do get better... I got better.

—AGE 17

It Was Like Looking at a Life
I No Longer Had

During my junior year it seemed that things could not get any better. I had just gotten back together with my boyfriend, and my friends and I were closer than ever. It seemed that the four of us couldn't be any closer. I had a particular girl that I was really close to. We always had the same activities, and anywhere I was, she was there, too.

My high school contains only juniors and seniors, and when we became juniors for some reason all of the seniors didn't like her. While her other so-called "friends" would agree behind her back with everything the seniors would say about her, I stuck up for her. It was just like that . . . or so I thought.

In February we had a big snow one weekend that stuck around and got us out of school for two days. Basically out of nowhere no one called me. It may not sound like that big of a deal, but when you spend every minute with these girls and all of the sudden they don't call you or answer your calls you start to wonder.

I had talked to one of my guy friends and he said

that he had hung out with the girls all weekend. The whole situation snowballed, and they all treated me as if I didn't even exist. It hurts so bad to know that these girls you have stood up for all these times, especially the one I mentioned earlier, could do that to you. I would go to school and they wouldn't talk to me. I would have to go to lunch by myself. It seemed like these girls had taken my life from me. I couldn't understand how anyone could do this, especially to a "friend."

To this day they don't see that they did anything wrong. They think the reason we didn't talk for four months was my fault. The day I came back to school after that long weekend without talking to any of them, they seemed to ignore me. My friend, Hillary, had a packet of pictures in her hand and I asked to look at them. She seemed hesitant and said they were no big deal, but she still gave them to me. Inside were pictures of the three other girls playing in the snow at a friend named Brian's house, and inside playing poker with the boys.

Before I saw the pictures I had asked her why no one called me that weekend and what they did. She said they didn't really do anything and that they just all hung out at each others' houses. Because they all live in the same neighborhood, they didn't call because they didn't think that I could drive in the snow....

Things just seemed to escalate. They stopped waiting for me to go to lunch with them, stopped calling me on the weekends. You know how girls sometimes give themselves and their group a nickname? They made whole new ones that did not include me.

I was devastated. In my high school you're friends with everyone, but you have your group of girls that you travel around with. I felt completely alone and isolated from everyone. Even my family tried to console me, but I still felt completely alone. I cannot even come close to describing how hurt I felt. I constantly had this physical tearing feeling in my heart.

My room is covered in pictures, drawings, collages, posters we had made together, inside jokes, traded clothes, knickknacks from trips we had all taken together, and every time I looked at them it was like looking at a life that I no longer had. I don't understand how people can be so cruel and not even realize it.

For about two months this went on. I didn't talk to ONE of them. They would always be together in the halls and I would be alone. I would pass right in front of them and they would not even acknowledge my presence. And I felt like when I passed, they would just laugh at me because I was always alone at lunch and in the halls. All I did was hang out with my boyfriend, and sometimes he would skip one of his classes and drive to my school to take me to lunch. He was the only person who could console me and somewhat make me understand that there was nothing wrong with me.

It wasn't until prom that they talked to me. They never even really apologized; they just tried to act like nothing happened. I was so bitter and full of resentment. Things between all of us weren't really cool on the surface until I started my senior year and decided that I wasn't going to spend it alone.

As far as their side of the story goes, I never really got it. One of the girls acts like she did nothing wrong and just went along with the other two girls. She also told me that Hillary said that she didn't do anything wrong.

I always asked what I did and no one would tell me. But thinking back on that time in my life, I remember one time about two weeks before this started we were all four in the car on a Friday night, and they all just started to pick me apart and tell me everything they didn't like about me. They said things that you should never ever say to someone that you call a friend, much less your best friend.

Hillary's reason was that her mom didn't want us hanging out anymore, but I don't think that that's true. I think it was hard as well to be friends with me when I was still with Kevin, because my boyfriend and hers were best friends and this guy was her first for everything. He was her first love, he took her virginity, he told her everything that she wanted to hear and then dropped her because he was going to college. So I think that it was hard for her to be around me when Kevin and I were still together, but that's just a theory.

I know that these girls think of it as just another fight that we had, and don't really understand how bad it messed me up. I don't trust girls now, and I don't trust my "friends."

All I have ever wanted was a best friend, the type you see on *Oprah* that are forty-five and still like sisters. Maybe someday I'll find a girl who I can trust, but I found out that girls at this age are mean, malicious, and liars.

—AGE 18

Please . . . Listen to My Cries

I don't know what's going on
I can't tell which way to go
I am so lost and confused
You don't even know.

My mind is such a mess
I don't know what to do
I need some way out
I wish that somebody knew.

I cry for help all the time
And wish that someone would care
This pain and confusion I have,
It is just too hard to bear.

Someone please help me
Before it is too late
I need someone's care and love
Please help me, don't wait.

—AGE 17

The Sound of Silence

When your friends turn on you, there's not much you can do except wait it out.

It usually happens like a thunderstorm. The sky is beautiful and blue, and without warning it turns black. The storm thrashes and booms, then the sun comes out again. Similarly, your friends need to get the anger out of their systems. I have heard many, many stories of girls who get totally annihilated by their friends, and then, out of nowhere, they walk up to her and say, "Hey, we're sorry about before. Can you come out this weekend?" The formerly rejected girl is like, "Hello? What?" (And her mom goes nuts, having vowed never to allow her precious girl to see those horrible creatures ever again.)

But that's not much help at this moment. What do you do right now?

Every three days, try to talk to the person who is controlling the group's anger. If there's more than one, approach each person, one at a time. Girls get their negative power from the support of others; that's why they're often nicer one-on-one. Do not talk to her on-line (see more about this on page 144).

Go up to her in the hallway, bathroom, lunch-room, or parking lot. Look her in the eye and keep your voice calm. Try not to cry. Tell her you want to know why she's upset, and that you want to apologize if you've done anything wrong. Tell her you're upset, too, and that you'll do what it takes to make things right. If she walks away, wait three days and try again.

Find someone else to hang with. Don't stand there in the hall or sit at lunch staring longingly at your friends. It will just provoke them to act like they are having the greatest time ever in your absence. Once you find someone else to talk with, don't act like *you* are having the greatest time ever in *their* absence. That will only make your friends angrier.

Don't try to replace your old friends with new people. Even if you're wishing every girl in your old group comes back in her next lifetime as a flea, that's your hurt and anger talking. When the day comes that you make up with them, you'll probably end up spending less time with or, let's face it, even ditching the new people you found. Is that okay? Not really, but it's what happens in these situations.

You owe it to any new friend you make not to make any promises you can't keep. If you end up adoring her and think you've found your soul mate, great; but be honest with yourself about what you'd do if you could have your old friends back. You have to consider your new friend's feelings and recognize that by ditching her you'd be doing what people are doing to you right now. If you end up being rude to her once you're back in good graces with your old group, you are turning on your new friend the same way your old ones turned on you.

You may be waiting for this hell to end, or you may have decided to move on; either way, you're going to need some positive energy in your life. Add something new to your day—sports, working out, a club, volunteering, a job, a class, maybe a hobby. Get obsessed with eighties movies or Harry Potter or an online community. Crochet. Do something. It'll take your mind off your temporarily lousy life, and you'll get to meet new friends in the process.

You feel terrible. Talk to someone about it: a parent, relative, teacher, mentor, social worker, psychologist, or guidance counselor. It helps to get your feelings out and have someone listen who won't judge you.

Keep a journal. I did when I was younger, and there were many times when it was the only "person" I had to talk to. A journal helped me organize my thoughts in a new way. It led me to deep insights about my relationships and new conclusions about myself.

Get online and become part of a teen cybercommunity. Join some list-servs and groups, or a chat room. Check out *www.gurl.com* or find a cool teen e-zine. I have learned from experience that when you're lonely, you can find good company in the strangest places.

Keep perspective. You are hurting, you are scared, you feel alone, but this will not go on forever. *Believe me.* Misery will not be the only thing you ever know. And as you can see from the authors in this book, there are silver linings to the clouds, although it may take a while to find them. Cry and scream and freak out, but remember: This will end, and your life will be rich and pleasurable and long...long beyond the girls who are bugging out on you.

If it gets really, really bad, see your guidance counselor or ask your parents about seeing a therapist. These situations have led many girls to develop clinical depression, anxiety, and other serious problems. Don't underestimate your feelings. We may live in a world that says girl bullying is no big deal, but you don't have to listen. Get help if you need it. All you have to do is ask.

Consider changing schools if you can. This is appropriate only in extreme circumstances. I have never met a girl who switched schools and wasn't happy she did. It's a chance to start over with a whole new set of people. If your thunderstorm seems like it will last forever, it may be just what you need.

Losing Trust

"I'm not friends with girls. Most of my friends are guys. They don't stab you in the back. With guys there's no drama. It's less complicated."

I've heard more girls than I can count say things like this. When girls break your heart, running away feels right. Even becoming a loner feels better than getting hurt again. Although it may not seem like a big deal right now, abandoning all hope of friendship with females is one of the biggest mistakes you can make in your life.

I'm not saying it doesn't make sense to feel that way. One of the first lessons you learn as a little kid is how to be friends with someone. You learn that if you're nice to someone, they'll be nice back. When your friends turn on you without warning or reason, it blows that lesson to smithereens. When one day you have an amazing group of friends and the next day no one speaks to you or tells you why, how are you supposed to ever trust anyone again?

First of all, it's rare for girls to be victimized by their friends more than once. Every girl I interviewed who changed schools as a result of being bullied said she was much happier, even popular, in a new place. When girls hurt each other that severely, it's usually the result of a long buildup of specific problems that won't be repeated in another situation.

Second, you may not realize it now, but when someone hurts you, you learn things—about people and yourself. You're going to get better at checking out new friends and picking the nice ones to keep close. That's one of the few good things about pain.

Take your time when you meet new people. There's

no rush. Deep scars have to heal. But if you stay convinced girls will hurt you, it's like opening your wound again and again. For if you forget about girls for good, you allow the ones who hurt you to win. You deprive yourself of a lifetime of girls' nights out, ya-ya sisterhoods, late night phone calls, and the amazing rush you get when you look at the person who is your best friend and know she feels exactly the same way. One of the ways to triumph over your turmoil is by leading a normal life of healthy intimacy with other girls.

Avoid other girls and you'll feel the loss in more than just your friendships. You'll also hurt yourself as a future leader. Ever hear of the Old Boys' Network? It's a system of older men helping younger guys move up the ladder of success, and it's one of the biggest reasons women still fall behind men at the highest levels of power. Women have to create networks, too. Experienced women have to take younger women under their wings, and girls have to seek out mentors. If you scorn girls in your social life, you're not going to walk into the office one day and suddenly be able to forge positive relationships with female colleagues and superiors.

Trust is a confusing thing in female friendships. The best and worst part of girls is how fast we can fall—yes, for each other. Think about it: It's very romantic, not in a sexual way, but in that fairy tale, we're-meant-for-each-other-and-will-be-together-forever kind of way. Finding your best friend is like having a light turned on inside you. You close your eyes and jump, and most of the time, it's the most amazing kind of free fall.

When I was on the *Oprah* show, a young woman in the audience told me about being hurt so severely by girls that she feared she could never trust anyone again. She felt she had no choice but to protect herself fiercely.

I told her this: Trust is something you build gradually with another person. You can't fall into friendship with someone until she's proved herself to you as a friend, and that comes only with time.

When you're ready, try this: If you've found someone you think you may want to be closer to, tell her a little secret, one you could live with becoming public. See what happens. If the secret gets back to you—if she told someone—you know she's not a good friend. You can walk away, or pull back relatively unharmed.

Intimacy with other females is one of life's most wonderful treasures. The beauty of the human spirit is its ability to regenerate, even in the face of risk: We hurt, recover, and want to try again no matter how much pain we feel. Yet healthy intimacy with someone is also very hard work; it's something you build, piece by piece, day by day. With patience and faith, you will find closeness with a girl who will earn your trust.

"IT'S THE WAY GIRLS SURVIVE"

Aggression, Fear, and Revenge

In this section, writers explore the darker side of girlhood and themselves. I applaud their courage. When you grow up in a world that asks you to be nice all the time, admitting that you're not, or that you've acted in ways you regret, is a risk.

These girls write about transformations: A girl goes from riches to rags when a queen bee gets her just desserts; from victim to bully when a girl makes the decision to turn her own pain into someone else's; and from witness to bystander when a girl becomes a "bully by association."

People brush off girl bullying as a "phase" or "girls being girls" because so many girls hide their ability to hurt others. Girls reach for the impossible ideal of being nice 24/7. They're quick to say they've been victims, that they're nice, that they'd never do anything terrible like those other mean girls.

Because girls are taught that expressing anger directly is wrong, many girls (and women) have no choice but to resort to secret acts of meanness. They project an image of themselves that others think is "fake." These "nice" girls separate themselves vehemently from those who have dared to show aggression, calling them bitches and skanks. They turn "mean" girls into unfeeling monsters, rather than the human beings they really are. When "good" girls deny their own anger and punish the ones who don't, they empower the culture that is forcing them to be nice all the time.

By coming forward with their stories, these brave writers show us that the aggressors, as much as their victims, are in need of our attention, help, and compassion. These girls provide the best proof yet that girls' aggression is more than a "rite of passage," and that really good girls aren't always so nice.

I Was My Own Worst Nightmare

People think it is something one "gets over," but believe me, it's not. I was bullied in junior high and it is an experience that still affects the person I am today. It is something that will always be a part of me and something I will never forget. I really don't think I could ever forgive those girls that made my life miserable.

I was bullied, and then became the aggressor later on in life. In junior high I attended a small, upscale, private school in the Midwest. Unlike larger public schools, we had small classes of about twenty or so people. Few new kids came to our school and few kids left. It was always the same kids in the same classes, all of us together, and I believe this was a recipe for trouble.

I wasn't like the other girls. I was tall, thicker than most of the other girls. My family didn't have very much money, while the other girls came from wealthy families. My relationships with the girls were very hot and cold. One minute we were all the best of friends, but at any moment, the girls would turn on someone, usually me, and I would be completely alone.

Being in such a small school, when one girl hated you, all of the girls hated you, and most of the boys went along with it. And it wasn't just the grade I was in that hated me; the grades both above and below me would despise me as well. More often than not, I wouldn't even know why the girls were angry with me. But sometimes it would be a complete betrayal.

I would say something to one of the girls, usually the one I was closest to at the time. I would say something to her in confidence, and because she wanted to be popular, she would run to another girl, stab me in the back, and tell that other girl what I had said.

The result was a snowball effect, until finally what I had said had been changed so much. One time, I was so upset and so tired of being bullied and ignored that I called my grandmother and asked her to pick me up from school. I just couldn't handle it anymore. I was sick of being alone. I was sick of eating lunch by myself. I was sick of fighting back tears and I was sick of being told by teachers to just ignore the other girls. They made it sound so easy, but how can you ignore an entire class of girls calling you names?

Once out of middle school I thought things would be different, but they weren't. My first year of high school, I attended an all girls' private school. My first few months were great. I made a lot of friends and for once I felt popular and happy with who I was. But I made one false move, and everything changed for me.

I began dating a guy another girl had a crush on. I barely knew the girl and had no idea she had feelings for this boy. When I broke up with him, she started vicious rumors about me and somehow managed to "steal" all of my friends from me. It was slowly at first, a few calls not returned, a few dirty looks. But within a few weeks it escalated into a full-blown showdown during lunch. All thirteen girls ganged up on me at our lunch table, accusing me of saying things I had never said. They called me everything from a liar to a slut.

Soon, I had no friends. I sat alone at lunch. I skipped classes just so I didn't have to face any of those girls and the looks they would give me. My grades dropped dramatically. Finally, I made the decision to transfer to a public school to escape the girls and the torment. I found solace in the fact that I would be going to a new school where I knew no one. It was a chance to start over. I vowed to make a change. I did make a change, but not for the better.

At my new high school, I became the bully. I talked badly about girls behind their backs. I even made a few girls cry in the hallways before classes. I prided myself on being popular and in charge. No one messed with me because they knew if they did I could turn everyone that "mattered" in the school against them in no time. I was downright cruel.

For me, it was a defense mechanism. I thought if I pretended to be strong, and if I picked on everyone else that was weaker than me, no one would see the chubby girl that was tortured just years earlier. I felt as long as I was making fun of someone else, they couldn't turn the tables and make fun of me. I had the "better-them-than-me" mentality.

It wasn't until my senior year in high school that I realized exactly what I was doing. While at the mall one evening I ran into a girl that had gone to my high school my sophomore year. I recognized her face but couldn't quite remember her name. She was tall, thin, and very pretty, so I assumed I must have been friends with her, considering my elitist and shallow attitude.

I approached her, said hello, and began making small talk. She had a look of sheer terror on her face as I talked to her.

Finally she spoke up and said, "You have no idea who I am, do you?"

I confessed that I recognized her face but couldn't remember her name.

"I'm Monica Taylor," she replied, and I knew why she had a look of disgust and horror on her face.

I had made Monica's life miserable for an entire year. I had convinced boys to make mooing sounds when she walked past them in the hallway, I laughed as my friends sat back and threw food at her during lunch, I called her everything from pig to fat and laughed as I did it. I was awful to this girl.

I was absolutely speechless and felt complete remorse when she started to cry and told me that she had had to move away because I had made her life so miserable. She revealed that her weight loss was due to an eating disorder that I directly contributed to by making fun of her weight. Her final words to me were, "You are a nasty person."

With that she walked away, and I was left with the horrible realization that I had become the very type of person I hated. I was my own worst nightmare.

From that point on, I vowed to be a different person. I promised myself I would no longer make fun of people, for any reason. I couldn't make people feel as badly as people had made me feel in the past. I didn't have that right.

Making the change wasn't easy. The habit of ridiculing others was almost second nature to me. I was forced to cut ties with most of my so-called friends. I refused to spend time with people that picked on others. It resulted in a lot of backlash for me, but I came to understand that people like that weren't worth my time or effort in the first place. I knew from experience that their hurtful words stemmed from their own insecurities, not mine.

I made a real effort to get to know people I wouldn't normally spend time with and found out how wonderful those people were. I made so many real friends. I knew these people wouldn't stab me in the back or talk bad about me when I wasn't around.

I apologized to everyone I had made fun of. This was the most difficult task for me. It meant I had to admit I was wrong. It meant I had to admit that they were bigger, better people than I was. But I knew it had to be done, not just for my own sanity, but because I knew I would feel so much better if those girls who had tortured me would only apologize.

My senior year, my year of change, was one of the best of my life. I made so many new friends and found out that you don't have to be mean and hurtful to have good friends. I was more popular being respectful and kind to others than I would have ever been had I stuck with being mean.

Those experiences have made all the difference in my life, and I am grateful that I was able to see the light and make a change for the better. I hope others can see the errors of their ways and do the same someday.

—AGE 21

Friend Trouble

I have a best friend who has been my friend since fourth grade. I am now in fifth grade. Last year she was the only person, friend-wise, who I could depend on. I did have another best friend, but she had moved away. I really missed her, and I counted on my other best friend to make up for that loss. She did. For a while.

At the end of fourth grade, we made another friend. She was really nice, or at least, I thought so. We really liked her, so we really bonded with her. We became the best of friends. We played with each other a lot, and I was so happy. I thought that now, with two friends to depend on, I would feel somewhat better about my friend moving away. And I did. For a while. Now here came summer. We said good-bye, and vowed to always be friends.

Here comes fifth grade. As luck would have it, each of us are in different classes. We don't let that affect our friendship. *Oh no.* We played with each other and talked to each other every chance we got.

Anyway, we made up this new game during recess, when we would all go down the slides backward, holding each others' feet. This was fun. For a while. Now, this became a problem. The problem with this game was that it was really fun, but it also hurt the person that went first. And the friend that we had made in fourth grade was a little chubby, so we always made her go first. She didn't mind this. For a while.

Soon, she began to ask why she always had to go first. We couldn't tell her that we made her go first because she was fat, so we avoided the question.

Finally, she said that I had to go first. I'm average fat. I couldn't make my other best friend go first, because she's as skinny as a skeleton. So I agreed to go just once. It hurt as much as I thought it would and a little more. I didn't want to do that again.

When we got back to the top of the slides, she told me that I had to go first again. I refused, and she asked why. I burst out, "Because you're fat and you will crush me!"

Well, that really offended her, and she went away crying. She is spoiled rotten. She came back after a while, sat down next to me and my best friend, and said she was sorry. I did, too, and I really meant it. Then the next day, she told me I had to go first again. I said no. She told me this every day. My best friend didn't have to go first because she is too skinny.

Finally, one day, I got so mad at her, I pushed her.

She almost fell over a railing onto the ground. She pushed me back and we started kicking and punching each other. She knocked my glasses off, and I kept hitting her face. Finally she pulled away and said, "THAT HURT!" She went down the slide and sat at the bottom crying. I sat down at the top, and started crying, too.

My other friend didn't take sides. She kept going between me and my fat friend and talking to each of us. My friend came back up and my fat friend came up with her. We both apologized, but we didn't mean it. Ever since then, me and my fat friend both try to hang out with my skinny friend.

Here is the problem. My skinny friend has divorced parents and is not really dependable. You don't know who's at her house when. My parents wouldn't let me sleep over at her house for this reason, so me and my skinny friend did not have any fat friend free time.

By this time, my skinny friend didn't like my fat friend either. We tried to drop hints, like ignoring her, but they didn't work. We had bonded too much with her.

Finally, we decided to do a three-way phone call and tell my fat friend that we didn't want to be friends with her anymore. We did this and immediately hung up. My fat friend's mom called my skinny friend's mom because she didn't know my number, and my skinny friend got in trouble. My fat friend was crying.

She's just not getting it and I guess we'll have to live with it. We just can't tell her, or she'll tell the teacher. We're thinking what to do, and until then I guess she still thinks that we're best friends!

—AGE 11

My Shameful Story of Victimization, Paranoia, and Redemption

At first, when I would hear stories of girls ruining other girls' lives in horrible backstabbing stunts, I would deny that it could have ever happened in my school among my fellow students. I went to a private Catholic school where almost everyone had known each other since kindergarten, and where girls made up barely over one-third of the grade.

But I was wrong; it was one year ago that I realized this horrible fact. Two years ago my very best friend of three years moved halfway across the country. For a while we made it work, but that summer I went to visit her and we realized that we had nothing in common anymore. We haven't spoken since July 2002.

So I go into seventh grade, into a bunch of girls with well-established and defined groups of friends. What the hell am I supposed to do? This is when I realize how badly other girls had psychologically hurt me throughout my short life. Every time someone that I had approached with friendship talked to someone else I became unrealistically paranoid that my proposal was the conversation topic they found so funny. I literally trusted no one. I was alone and miserable, but what hurt even more than the insane paranoia was that my own mother could look into my eyes and have no idea how much pain I was in.

So after I spend a couple months loathing my life and my best friend, for leaving, I approached two girls I had known since I was five. Being separate from other people anyway, they accepted my proposal. I had friends, but I still couldn't fully trust them.

Well, the year goes by and I find myself becoming pretty good friends with multiple members of the "popular" group, which is nice. So I start hanging out with them and am invited to parties. Life, though I continue to be paranoid about everything that is happening, is pretty good.

Now enters the crazy unexpected plot twist. My best friend from ages three through seven begins to hang around me. I completely ignore the fact that we're in the same classes and jump right to the paranoid conclusion that she is using me to get to the "popular" girls.

Here is where I go from innocent victim to card-carrying member of the international "evil" girls' society. Now I begin to get upset that she thought she could do that to me. So every time she said anything about anyone in the grade, I made sure they knew what she said, and what she really meant by it. Pretty soon the whole grade started to see how annoying she was as well.

She never, from what I know, even considered that it was me giving her the bad rap. I think that because she never stopped hanging out with me. When I realized this, of course, my mission went from getting back at her, to getting her to leave me alone. She is not one who can take a hint, so the only way to get her to leave was to tell her to her face. As every girl knows, as soon as you do that you're labeled a bitch to everyone you know and their families.

So, here I am hating the only person who *really* wants to hang with me. The group I do hang with is made up of me, a pretty annoying guy, another girl, and her boyfriend, who happens to be one of the two guys I'm in love with (the other one is another of my best guy friends), and neither like me. On top of that, I can't tell anyone in fear that my mother might find out, which would mean I would have to talk to her, which, believe me, is impossible, and this is my life at least until high school. So basically my life would suck even if I weren't paranoid.

—AGE 14

Looking for Someone to Dominate

It started freshman year and I was fourteen. My first few months of school were basically me trying to find some group of girls to fit in. I go to an all-girls' school, which could be either really easy or extremely hard. I tried hanging out with a few girls I'd met but they didn't seem to fit with me. And then later I found the group I fit into perfectly.

That's when I started looking. Looking for someone to dominate. Because when you're a freshman, everyone else seems to dominate over you but if I could just find someone weaker than myself, I would have that much more power.

And then I found my target. Jodie. At first I hadn't really noticed her, but then I heard a rumor that she was talking about me behind my back. And that's what set me off.

She had just enough guts to talk about me but not enough friends to back her up. And so I told all my friends about her and what she may or may not have said. I worked it so my best friend hated her, too, and

122

would try and intimidate her in the halls during school. Even in P.E. I would rag on her. That's the perfect place to really intimidate someone. That's where I could get more physical while whispering vicious things to her and fighting over a puck in hockey. I could pin her against the wall or "accidentally" hit her with my hockey stick.

One day I didn't know where the hockey puck was, and she yelled back at me that she had it. But she did it with sarcasm in her voice and that just didn't fly with me. I yelled back, "Bite me!!" With a few other choice words, of course. And then she cowered and never said anything to me again.

When walking down the halls I would seek her out in order to bump into her and say something sarcastic yet equally vicious. Or even just a glare in the hallway to make sure she remembered who was dominating who.

At the end of the day, my best friend Lori would come back and explain to me how she intimidated her in one of her classes. It was great. I felt powerful. And most of all, important.

My friends knew I did it, but I don't think the teachers did. How could they know without her telling them? And I never got called into the office because I never hurt her — physically that is. They didn't know I was trying to make her life hell.

Needless to say she doesn't go to my school anymore. And honestly, I was disappointed to hear she wasn't coming back the following year. Even now I look for people who I can dominate. People who I can get others to hate or at least be annoyed with. I know it's a bad habit, but it's a habit that's hard to kick. It's the way girls survive with other girls. By either undermining them or otherwise. Ironically, it seems to be how we get along.

—AGE 17

I Just Stood By and Let It Happen

I can't say I was a bully by the popular definition: I never beat anyone up, I never really verbally went all out on someone with curses and all. But I know I've hurt people. I mastered the silent treatment. I've been a bully through gossip and in doing so I've really damaged someone's reputation.

I hate to admit it, but I'm the kind of girl where I don't want to sit next to the loser girl or the outcast. If I talked to the loser girl and if I'm seen hanging out with her, my own reputation could be damaged. The people I've managed to become "in" with would think I was uncool.

I was the bully in a group — a collective bully. I was a bully in the sense that I would hang out with my louder friends when we all confronted someone we didn't like. I was a bully by association. I never really did the verbal confrontation myself. I just stood by and let it happen.

I remember there was this girl Erica who I was friends with. She wasn't exactly the most popular girl in school. I sat next to her in algebra class, and we learned to crack jokes. I even learned to enjoy sitting with her.

This girl Mary who I was friends with was cool — tough and popular. She didn't like the fact that I was talking to Erica, so she kept pestering me about my relationship with her. Mary was like, "Erica is a loser and so why do you keep talking to her?"

One day, I was hanging out with Mary and we walked past Erica's locker. But as we were passing, Mary started questioning Erica. She was like, "Who the hell do you think you are? I saw you checking out my boyfriend Mike!" and she shoved her backward. Erica just swallowed and as much I just wanted to stick up for her, I didn't.

Everyone was watching. Even Chris, the boy I liked, the most popular guy in school, was not too far away.

Erica said, "I'm sorry."

I was just so shocked! She hadn't even done anything wrong and she was apologizing to Mary. I know Mary made up the whole scenario just to put me in a weird position and to let Erica know her place. I knew it was cruel.

Looking back, now that I'm more independent, I know I should have stood up for Erica. Screw Mary. Yet I knew I hurt Erica. We never talked again. I was a bully by association. A bully of the masses. I know I'm not like that anymore and considering the fact that I have been bullied by other girls, I don't like really thinking about the fact that I've been on the wrong side. This is actually the first time I'm mentioning it. Maybe I can help someone by telling this story. Maybe I won't. At least I'm being honest.

—AGE 16

Harmless Fun

When I was in fifth grade, I moved to a new school with a lot of my friends. In the first week, I sat down at a random seat and it turned out to be someone else's. This girl that it belonged to said something along the lines of, "That's my seat, get out of it now."

I said something like, "No, I don't see your name on it."

Then she said, "Get off or I'll give you one of these." She grabbed me by the collar of my shirt and pulled it so I was forced to get up. I walked away. I never ever forgot that moment, but I never confronted her about it either. So as the year passed, I began to dislike everything she did. I hated her.

In sixth grade, I hung out with the more "outgoing" group. The girl that "picked on" me in fifth grade was in the other group. None of my friends liked her. It wasn't that she did something horrible to us all. It was just a thing. Anyway, as we got older, my distrust of her and hatred for her grew. Every year, our class got smaller and smaller. We got to know each other more, but I still didn't like her.

We used to get onto a fake screen name and start talking to her crushes, saying that it was her. We made the guys think that she was a complete freak and stalker. It was fun, and I didn't feel any guilt. I mean, she picked on me first, right? (That's what I thought then.)

In eighth grade, we went on a class trip to New York City. Nobody wanted to room with her because she was weird. She smelled like fish, and she was always home-sick, so she'd whine about it. Nobody wanted to hear about that.

So throughout the trip we took turns taking her. It was like a punishment. She was very into Wicca. Well, not Wicca, but more like witches. It wasn't Wicca...it was weird...anyway, me and my other two friends decided to mess around with her 'cause it'd be fun.

We decided to become "witches." We would pretend to "talk" to each other mentally in class when everything was prompted. We even made it look like we made things appear from the sky. It freaked her out and I enjoyed that, too.

Besides that we did other little "harmless" stuff, like make up rumors and whine to teachers. We even cried about her to make it seem like she was horrible. She wasn't really horrible; I think that my hatred just grew the more I kept it in. She still doesn't know why I was so mean to her. Looking back on all the things I did, planned, and participated in, I do regret it, because she was a really nice person at heart. She just lied sometimes.

I'm in tenth grade now, and we go to totally different schools. I still talk to her. The only time she IMs me, though, is when she wants to talk about guys. No offense or anything, but I go to an all-girls' school, and I hear enough "I don't get guys" stories. But I play nice and help her through it because that's what friends are for. I mean, I can tell her I don't really care, but it doesn't annoy me, so I don't have to.

—AGE 15

Follow the Leader

Waking up to an alarm clock is not half as refreshing as being awoken by the scent of the summer breeze. It is so aggravating for the alarm clock to interrupt the pleasant dreams that keep you away from the stressful real world. Eventually, I always awaken. The aroma of pencil shavings and uncapped Magic Markers fill my room. I sit up gradually on the side of my bed; with another slight move I might fall face first onto the carpeted floor.

I glimpse over my shoulder at the blinking clock — it is almost time for school. Yet another day of seventh grade. My excitement is overwhelming, ugh.

"*Briiinnng, briiiinnng,*" the uneasy sound of the telephone breaks the silence.

"Leslie!!" By the tone of the goody-two-shoes voice on the other end, I knew it was Rebecca.

"Hey Bec, what's up?" I reply as I rub my eyes, hoping to keep them opened.

"Just calling to remind you to bring the tank top that I left at your house to school today." I agree and tell her I will see her soon. She came over during the weekend with my two other good friends, Kayla and Zoe. I did not invite any other girls from school; I don't usually invite the other girls anywhere, to be perfectly honest.

The moment I step onto the school's property, my mood changes drastically. From the time I hop out of bed, to the time I devour my breakfast, I am the most petulant person to be around. When I am in the presence of my friends, there is not one moment my face looks despondent. I walk proudly toward the cluster of my girlfriends, and we start teasing people about anything that we are capable of teasing them about. The bell rings loud enough for people in the next town over to hear—that is one of the things on our school's repair list. Kayla, Zoe, Rebecca, and I run toward the building; we break away from the gathering of our friends so we can gossip alone.

As the year went on, my three good friends and I never spent much time with the other girls. We kept to ourselves. Zoe and Rebecca became awfully close, as did Kayla and I. My and Kayla's friendship became stronger every day. From babysitting together, and trips to my grandmother's house, to skiing, we were inseparable. Every Friday, the four of us would hang out at one of our houses. Despite the fact that invitations to the other girls' houses were always on the table, we hardly ever accepted them. We enjoyed the company of ourselves, and ourselves only.

Classes were brutal. The ninth-period bell was the solitary fixation that separated my captive hours from my freedom. Eventually, it would ring and I would dash to my locker. The hallways were crowded; always are, always will be. As I walked through the long narrow hallway, I would tap all of the girls on the shoulder. Ahead of me, I had spotted Zoe. I greeted her and attempted to tell her about some kid farting in class, but she turned and walked away from me. Zoe and I have never really hit it off. We were friends by accident, you could say. But lately, we had grown closer than ever before, and to turn away from me struck me as odd.

Days turned into weeks and weeks turned into months: Zoe, plain and simple, did not like me any longer. Either she stared me down during school, or she just did not even notice me at all. Talking online was the closest I could get to Zoe. She never told me why she became so mad at me. She always referred back to "Leslie, you know what you did." Honestly, I haven't a clue of what I did to hurt her. While I was around her, I made sure I did not utter or do anything stupid. Zoe was the type of person that you *want* to be friends with. Her personality drives you toward her in a way that if she were mad at you, you would be on your knees for forgiveness. Every school has one of those kinds of girls.

Kayla and Zoe have been friends since elementary school. Because of Rebecca and me they never spend much alone time. Kayla stuck by me while Zoe despised me, which made her seem like the ideal friend. Even though each weekend Zoe would invite Kayla and Rebecca over, I would stay strong and try not to become upset by it. Zoe, Rebecca, and Kayla started hanging out with the other girls. Surprisingly, none of them invited me along.

The end of the year came, and I was so grateful I would be going off to camp soon enough. I had hoped that by the end of the year Zoe would have accepted my apologies, but she didn't. Throughout the year I must have apologized more than ten times to Zoe; I received no acceptance from her.

Rebecca started acting strange toward me. She never called to hang out with me and never acted enthusiastic online whenever I would talk to her. I was leaving for camp in one week, and I sat home alone the entire time. You could see Kayla's attitude change about me. I always was aware of the fact that Kayla did not have a backbone, that she was no leader, just a follower. I never expected her to leave my side though.

I invited Rebecca and Kayla to sleep at my house the night before I left for camp, and drive me up there, but Rebecca declined. I was brave enough to invite Zoe to accompany me as well. I should have expected the retort she gave me. Kayla accepted the invitation, which made me in high spirits. I thought this could be the foundation to starting over.

The day before I left, Rebecca, Kayla, and Zoe were together. They were at Zoe's house with some boys. I was at home, fixed on Zoe's away message. I can't remember what it said, only the last section of it. "Loveee — Zoe Kay and Bec."

My mind boggled about the actions of Kayla. I kept thinking why my name was *not* on that away message, why Kayla was *not* at my house, why they most likely were *not* even thinking of me at all. So many things to "not" do in one away message. My best friends have betrayed me, I was leaving for two months and they did not even have the decency to say good-bye.

As I sat in my room with tears rolling down my face, the doorbell rang. I knew nobody would answer it, aware of my family's lazy habits. I decided to clean my face off and go open the door. I looked out the window, and there stood Kayla with a large bag on her shoulder and massive sandals on her feet. I scurried toward the door and opened it with excitement. She came inside and I knew everything would be okay.

Summer went by so fast, like it always does. A summer with many letters full of "I miss you" and "come home soon." I wrote and received tons of letters to and from Kayla. I gathered four letters from Rebecca and wrote her at least twice. I also wrote some letters to the other girls, and I built up my courage and wrote to Zoe. Zoe never wrote back.

Once again school started. This time I was not so excited for it to begin. My car pool picked me up as usual. Rebecca is in that car pool; she did not pass me a second glance. I stepped onto the school's property, this time not so proud. Everyone hugged one another, and shared quick stories of their summer. Nobody hugged me. Nobody told me a story. I walked toward Kayla, hoping to find someone who would actually be excited to see me. Kayla looked at me in a way I will never forget. That one solitary look said it all. It told me to not go near her, I would embarrass her, or she was not allowed to talk to me anymore. I headed over to some of the other girls, feeling a little abandoned. The girls did not care to see me; they did not miss me at all. I walked into school alone.

The school year went on, Rebecca took me off of her profile. Kayla eventually decided to have no profile, most likely because she did not want me to know what was going on. I walked in the hallways alone, from class to class. I looked at all of my other friends I never hung out with. I realize I got what was coming to me.

I saw Kayla all the time in the hallways; she never looked at me, and when she did it was not a pleasant look at all. She forgets how good a friend I was to her, and I doubt she knows why she had so much hatred toward me. Rebecca was not very subtle with not liking me. She gave me looks that were so insinuating. You know the expression, "If looks could kill," well, let's just say if this statement was literal I would not be here to tell my story. Zoe and I never associated. We never looked at each other, never thought about each other, and never were aware of each other's existence. I was so lonely.

Zoe and Rebecca were the type of people that intimidate others. If they ostracized someone, the other girls followed. I had no friends in the entire school, and I hated it. After school, I would stand outside with nobody to talk to. The boys looked at me as though I had three eyes. I started to appreciate the people who I used to make fun of; it was not fair of me to do that to them. I only wanted one thing, and that was to go back in time and fix whatever I did to hurt Zoe. Zoe ruined my eighth grade year, and it is not even winter yet.

It has been four months since school has started, since my friends have left me, since I *wanted* the weekend to come. I have not had a lot of conversations with people at school, and I am getting used to that concept. My schedule during the day is simply to listen to the teachers and walk from class to class. There is nobody to walk with in the halls, but at least I get to class on time.

Another day of school rolls around; I wake up early for extra help in math. My dad drives me to school, and as I slam the door shut, I see Kayla. Kayla is right by the door, the only way to enter the building. I walk toward the front door with my head up high.

"Hey Les," a voice utters my name. I turn around and face my ex-best friend. A smile disembarked upon my face.

"Hey Kayla," I reply in a calm tone. I open the door and head to the math room. As I walk up the brightly painted stairwell, I remembered what my mom once told me, "Hurt me once, shame on you; hurt me twice, shame on me."

—AGE 13

Why Is She Acting Like This?

One of the most annoying things adults tell girls when someone's being mean to them is "she's just jealous."

Please.

When I'm talking to a parent, and she tells me what's happening to her cut-down and devastated daughter, and the parent says the other girl's just jealous, here is what I am thinking: So, Mrs. X, that really popular girl who's excluding Jess and talking about her behind her back and ruining her life is doing all of it out of a deep sense of wishing she could be more like Jess?

I'm sure Jess is so comforted by that.

The "she's-just-jealous" excuse has been around longer than panty hose, and it's been about as positive a contribution to girls' lives. The truth is that girls, like anyone else, get mean for any number of reasons. According to scientific research, kids may show aggression in school if they've got problems at home. Divorce, illness, addiction, death, financial trouble: Any of these can stress someone out to the point where they have to let go of a lot of negative energy at school, including fear.

Yes, fear. Not all mean girls operate out of a brute desire to hurt someone, although there are certainly some who do. Fear is often expressed as anger.

Imagine it: Your dad's been sick for a long time. There's no end in sight, no one has any time for you, you're freaking out about how your family's falling apart, and suddenly all your close relationships seem like they're in jeopardy. You start pushing people away because you're afraid of getting attached to them—they might leave you like your dad is about to—or maybe you're so angry at your messed-up life that you have no patience anymore, and the stupidest things you never cared about before are suddenly filling you with rage. It happens. In a situation like this, the most terrified girls can become pretty terrifying themselves.

Another reason girls get mean is "monkey see, monkey do." If you've got a mom who is manipulative, gossipy, and backstabbing, you've got a good chance of going down that road, too. Sometimes the moms actually urge their daughters to behave aggressively, and still others get involved in their daughters' fights like they were just another member of the clique. I've heard of plenty of moms who participate in e-mail and IM wars between their daughters' friends.

Some bullies hurt their friends through domination and control. Almost like stalkers, they monitor their friends' every move, demand their exclusive attention, and threaten them with abandonment or worse if they refuse to comply. In these cases, the "low self-esteem" explanation really does apply; the girl bullies operate out of a fear that no one would be their friends if given a choice in the matter.

To be sure, there are plenty of mean girls who really are jealous, or competitive, or threatened in some way by the strengths of another person. But there is no evidence whatsoever that jealousy is the big reason why girls act out. Aren't girls' lives a bit more complicated than that?

For thousands of years, women have been barred from showing aggression. Although most people never spoke of the darker side of females, jealousy seems to have been the exception. We have seen females vulnerable to jealous rages in stories ranging from Delilah in the Bible to Disney's Cinderella. Jealousy is the publicly acceptable way to explain female aggression.

But here's what a lot of people don't get: All women and girls get jealous, competitive, or threatened at different points in their lives, including the nicest people in the world. It's not the most terrible thing to happen, either. Jealousy is a totally natural, appropriate feeling to have in a world that places ridiculous pressure on kids to achieve, look good, and be popular.

Our culture tells girls to be nice all the time, so girls learn that jealousy and competition are "babyish," "selfish," and wrong. And if something's wrong, good girls had better hide it—just like they try to hide their other negative feelings. When the hottest guy in the grade asks the new girl out, and you get that weird feeling in the pit of your stomach, isn't it easier to blame her and say she's a slut? Think about it: Aren't the new girls at school who get cast as sluts or bitches or full-of-themselves usually pretty, self-confident, and liked by guys? Isn't the girl who constantly puts her "best friend" down in front of guys and chirps "Just kidding!" when her friend gets offended really just insecure?

I'm not innocent. On my good days, I'm willing to admit that I'm jealous of Gwyneth Paltrow, but find me on a day I feel like a slug and I am all, "Gwyneth Paltrow is so annoying. She is not even pretty." Cue eye roll, weird nasal noise.

Jealousy is one of many reasons why girls act out, but it is not the end-all, be-all. If girls talked honestly about what they were jealous of, we'd see a lot fewer explosions of rage. As with anger, the question is not whether or not you're going to get jealous, but how you're going to handle those feelings.

Are You Mad at Me?

Let's say you and I are friends. The bell's about to ring for first period, and you're cramming for a Spanish quiz. You're walking to class, half scanning your notes and half trying to make sure you don't trip and fall. I walk by and say, "Hey!"

You don't respond. I wheel my head around to watch you walk down the hall, a sinking feeling in my stomach. Why are you ignoring me? Why are you mad? I slide into my chair during first period and start to think. It must be this. It must be that. I can't concentrate. I'm freaking out. By the time the bell rings, I've got at least three different reasons why you must be mad, and the more I think about it, the angrier I am getting at you.

What's going on? Girls struggle to express their anger, so they often use body language like the silent treatment to express their feelings. But when silence equals anger, signals can get crossed; if someone accidentally doesn't respond to you—like when you say hi, or in a conversation—you may wrongly translate her silence to mean anger. Girls end up drawing big conclusions based on very little information. They get "paranoid," assuming the worst scenario when many other possibilities exist. The more they think, the more they wonder, the more scared they get. As a result, conflicts develop for no reason.

The next time you think someone's ignoring you, try not freaking out unless it happens again. It's worth the wait. It will save you a huge amount of anxiety. Find the person you think is angry, say hi, and if she says hi back, you're cool. If you need more reassurance, ask her directly if she's okay or if things are okay between the two of you.

If you decide to tell her why you're asking, don't be

surprised if she gets annoyed. A lot of girls I interviewed felt frustrated that they had to say hi all the
time to everyone they knew. Try to remember it's not
personal. Even if they don't exactly say it, they are annoyed at the world that forces them to be a smiley,
superfriendly girly-girl, even when they don't feel like
it, and punishes them with people getting mad at them
when they're not.

IM and E-mail:
Clicking Your Way through a Fight

Let's say you feel like a friend of yours has been weird
to you all day. You think maybe she's ignoring you, but
you're not sure. You want to ask her about it, but you
can't really find the right moment, and anyway, you're
kind of nervous about what she might say. All day
you're sitting in class thinking about it, watching her
pass notes with someone else and wondering if she's
writing about you. She comes late to lunch and doesn't
sit next to you. After that, you're not even sure what
happened. There might have been a science quiz that
you wrote the answers to in Spanish.

By the time you get home, you know exactly what
you are going to do. You walk in the house, put your
bag down, grab a snack. You do the how-was-school-
honey-it-was-fine-but-did-anything-special-happen-no-
I-gotta-go-upstairs thing with your mom and get

online. Your friend is on. You grab the keyboard, click on her screen name and type:

"Are you mad at me?"

It begins. For the next thirty minutes, the two of you are furiously typing back and forth.

> YOU3456: *u really seem weird and i just want to know if i did anything to make u mad.*

> HER1234: *gawd don't worry stop being soooo sensitive!!!!!!!*

You sit in frozen silence, your fingertips tingling on the mouse, waiting.

Waiting.

> HER1234: *jk! :)*

The air in your lungs rushes out. You can breathe again.

Fighting on IM is a huge mistake. Girls know this but they do it anyway. Ironically, the same reasons girls think it's a good idea are actually the reasons why it's a terrible idea.

First, you can't see her face. This is good, you think, because you're afraid of saying something the wrong way. You're also nervous you might say something you don't mean. You're afraid she'll know you're angry at her. Now all you have to look at is a blinking box on a computer screen.

But when all you see is a blinking box, you don't know what *she* means. And you don't know when *she's* angry. Since you're already nervous and probably a little paranoid, in the split second you have to interpret what she writes and reply, you decide that she's attacking you. You write back something mean, and the temperature gets turned up. Meanwhile, she's about to type "jk" or never meant anything mean in the first place. Too late for you, though.

You can't hear her tone of voice. This is good, you think, because you don't have to experience her angry emotions. You can simply respond to the words on the screen. But you're nervous, even scared, about fighting. She says something like "stop being sensitive" and you totally lose it because you think it's the worst thing she's ever said to you. Unfortunately, you couldn't hear that she was just kidding.

You don't have to have the fight by yourself. This is good, you think, because you can have your best friend with you (in cyberspace, on the phone, or in person) while you're going through the drama. She can give you advice and support. But behind that blinking box, your "friend" could be three or four people cutting and pasting your conversation to three other people, who send it on to their friends, and so on. If you slip up and say something that offends one of them, you may be in trouble with many more people than the girl you're IMing.

The big myth is that you can control what you're

going to say online. Yet you can't see the person, hear her tone of voice, or be sure it's safe to talk to her, so you're more likely to say things impulsively and carelessly, or just make comments that are misunderstood. I've yet to meet a girl who hasn't pressed "send" and then clapped her hand over her mouth and said, "Omigod."

What can you do instead?

For one thing, stop using the Internet as a way to express yourself. That doesn't mean you should stop writing down your feelings, but back in the old days, there used to be a thing called a pen. When you take the time to form the letters in your own handwriting, and when it takes longer than a millisecond to tell someone how you feel, a strange thing happens. You take more care with what you're saying. You get more time to cool off. You get to seal the envelope, sleep on it, then tear it open the next day and rewrite it. Writing by hand is the real way to control what you're saying.

If you write better by typing, type the letter, then write it by hand. But if you e-mail it, you run the risk of having more than one person read it. You know what that could mean. If you must e-mail it, sleep on it, then read it again the next morning. I guarantee you will probably edit it. If you hit "send" right away, you'll likely wish you hadn't.

If someone wants to get into it with you online, tell her you would love to talk with her but not via computer. Tell her you'll talk on the phone, in person, or through letters. Remember: It takes two to fight online. Instead, tell her you're worried that you won't be able to say the right thing online, or that you're better in person. Emphasize how open you are to what she has to say.

Don't, don't, don't give out your password. Do you give out your locker combination? House key? Diary location? So why are you telling people how to break into your account? Because that's what a lot of girls will do when they get mad. Angry girls will hijack your screen name and send e-mails and IMs to guys acting like they are you. They will subscribe you to porn sites. They will enroll you in crazy spam schemes. They will send notes to other girls about things you never said. You can avoid that risk entirely by keeping your password to yourself, or at least changing it when you get in a fight with someone.

IM and e-mail are like passing notes or writing on the bathroom wall. They are inadequate, impersonal tools of communication. When you have a problem with someone and need to resolve it, nothing will ever replace the experience of two open eyes and a firm, respectful voice.

Listening: The Most Important Part of Talking

When I wrote *Odd Girl Out* I spent a lot of time focusing on the trouble girls have voicing difficult feelings. The culture tells girls to be nice, and as a result, girls are fearful and anxious about conflict. They stay silent, get other girls to be on their side, or hold in their feelings until they explode with rage.

But what about the girls who do express their feelings? When they speak, what happens?

"They turn it around on me."

"They bring up all this stuff from like a month ago and then suddenly it's all *my* fault and *I* end up apologizing."

"They call me a bitch."

"They walk away."

The problem, I have learned, isn't just how we talk. It's also how we listen.

Ask yourself this question, and be honest: How do you feel when someone comes up to you with a serious look on her face and says, "Um, can I talk to you for a second?" You know something's up, and it's not going to be good. Here's how I generally feel: panicked, afraid, and most of all, defensive.

I get my claws up. I start wondering what she's going to say and how it's going to be wrong. By the time she opens her mouth to talk to me, I can barely hear her over the freaking out that's going on in my own head.

She says, "When you told Jess about my dad losing his job, I felt really angry."

I hear, "Boy, you have really messed up now. You are in huge trouble."

She says, "I told you that information was private."

I hear, "You really are a complete loser that screws up all the time. I can hardly believe I'm even friends with you. You totally suck."

She says, "It's really hard when I feel like I can't trust you, or that you're going to tell my secrets to someone."

I hear, "Seriously. I mean, why is anyone friends with you? I can't wait to tell everyone I know what you did."

This scenario is all too common among girls. The fear of direct conflict drowns out reason and common sense, giving us a warped translation of reality. Other girls hear just fine and simply deny what they've done or change the subject to justify their behavior.

Why do we do this? Here's one way of looking at it: If you're taught that being a good girl is the end-all, be-all of your girl life, the moment someone suggests you might have done something wrong is going to be a little nerve-racking. After all, the very center of your identity is threatened. It's no wonder many girls try so feverishly to deny they're anything but nice. Yet reacting with denial and defensiveness makes the situation worse. It makes the other person feel shut down, ignored, and invalidated. When the issue at hand cannot be discussed, the conflict escalates.

The next time someone tries to talk to you, try following some of these "rules of engagement."

Listen. In other words, don't talk. Let her say what

she needs to. Don't jump in with "But I...," or "Well, you..." Bite your lip, breathe deeply, do whatever it takes—but let her finish. You'll get your chance. Talking is most of what she needs to do.

Stay with the issue. This is the most important part of listening. If she wants to talk about A, don't respond by bringing up B. Whatever she has done in the past doesn't count. If she's angry because she feels like you're competing with her, don't bring up the fact that she was competitive with you last year, or even last month. Here's why bringing up other issues is almost always off-limits.

First, you're basically telling her that her feelings are invalid, she has no right to feel this way, and it doesn't matter what she thinks since there is clearly a reason why you were allowed to do what you did.

Second, you make the conflict bigger and harder to solve. A fight over one issue is clear; a fight over two or three or four starts to get tricky. If there is always a reason why someone acted poorly, then there is never a reason why anyone should ever apologize. If you were the one wanting an apology, would you agree?

Third, the more *issues* you bring into a fight, the more likely you will start to wonder about the *relationship* as a whole. It's sort of like this: "I thought we were just going to talk about this one thing, but we have so many problems, and the more we talk about them, the madder I get—I don't even understand why we bother being friends."

Fourth, the more issues you bring into a conflict, the more people you're likely to involve. Let's face it: Most fights between girls are not one-on-one. As you revive more incidents from the past, you run the risk of inviting other girls to get involved all over again. You may end up walking away from the friend you're fighting with and call up someone else who was involved in an earlier issue. "Oh my god, can you believe she has the nerve to tell me I'm doing *this* when remember how she did *that*? What*ever*!"

Finally, if you take the conflict away from the issue your friend needs to talk about, she will never really feel like you heard her. If she doesn't feel heard, she'll probably hold a grudge. And what's the thing girls hate most about their relationships with other girls?

"We never forget *anything. Ever.*"

If you don't feel listened to, you're certainly not going to forget, and why should you? If you respond to your friend's anger with three reasons why she really shouldn't be angry, or why she should be less angry, don't be surprised when she blows up at you the next time something small goes wrong.

I'm not saying you should lie down and nod dumbly to everything she says. You're allowed to explain your actions, especially what motivated you. But don't allow your fear of her anger, or of your friendship ending, to take over. If you let fear rule you, you will start justifying your behavior.

Apologize. And when you say you're sorry, mean you're sorry. Don't say, "I'm sorry you feel that way." That doesn't really mean anything except, "I'm sorry you're so sensitive that you have to get upset about such stupid things."

Try not to say, "I didn't mean to. I really didn't"— at least, not without saying you're sorry, too. Even if your intent was not to be aggressive, the effect was what hurt. That's ultimately what counts. After all, if you didn't mean to, I guess you didn't really do anything wrong. Isn't that what you're saying?

Say "I'm sorry." Period. Then press your lips together, no matter how hard it is, and be quiet. It's going to feel hard. So count to ten. Make a mental list of all the stuff you have to do. But stay quiet.

By following these rules, you have a good shot at a healthy conflict. But remember that in this situation someone has approached you; when you seek out someone to apologize to, they're not always ready to hear it.

Saying You're Sorry

When it comes to apologies, some people say "I'm sorry" as often as looking in the mirror—in other words, way too often—and others say it about as many times as Halley's comet comes, which is once every seventy-six years.

The girls who say "I'm sorry" all the time say the least about what happened to get them there in the first place. They say they're sorry as if it's a magic spell that will make all the bad feelings disappear. In reality, quick "I'm sorries" are Band-Aids. They may cover up the problem, but a grudge usually lingers. The friend who is annoyed today will be angry tomorrow.

Girls tell me all the time that "we fight over the *stupidest* things. We create drama over *nothing*." The "I'm sorry" girls are partly to blame. If you haven't talked a conflict through, but instead smooth it over with a breathless "I'm sorry," it's not going to take much to set your friend off next time. It could be something totally ridiculous, like the way you looked at her in the mirror this morning. Or the fact that you were loud in study hall. Doesn't matter: If she's angry to begin with, she'll be looking at you with dark goggles. Stuff that didn't bother her before is going to now.

The girls who don't apologize think saying you're sorry is about giving in, showing you're weak, and letting someone win.

"Win what?" I asked a group of girls.

"You know," they told me. "*Win*. The fight."

"But what do you lose if you say you're sorry?"

"You just *lose*."

"Lose what?"

"I don't know! You just do!" (This was usually followed by a really loud sigh, eye roll, or noise that's hard to spell out but kind of sounds like "*ach!*")

Although they don't say it, girls who rarely apologize are afraid of losing friendships, status, or both. After all, most conflicts between girls aren't taking place one-on-one; usually they're three-on-six, or nine-on-twelve, plus a few moms and people on your buddy list.

Many girls think saying they're sorry means the girl you're in a fight with—not to mention everyone on her side—has a right to drop you, dis you, or have power over you in some way. If you've got a posse on your side, you've got others to look out for besides yourself. If you "lose," they lose, too. That's a lot of pressure!

Here's what's wrong with this picture: Whether girls say they're sorry all the time or rarely, they both make the same mistake—they think a friendship conflict happens in black and white. One side wins and the other side loses. One side apologizes, the other side is apologized to. One of you is guilty, the other's not.

It'd be nice if things were that simple, but most of the time, they're just not.

In most cases, both of you have something to own, or take responsibility for. The stuff girls fight over is rarely black and white; there are always things two people interpret differently, or "shades of gray." It's rare that someone is completely innocent.

Even if you insist you did nothing, that you meant nothing, that it wasn't your intention to hurt her—that's not really the point. Sometimes you have to step back and ask yourself these questions:

- Do you love your friend? (That is, when she's not driving you crazy.)

- Do you care about how she feels?

- Do you want to keep being her friend in the long run?

If the answer is yes, it doesn't matter if you think you did nothing wrong. You can certainly explain that your intent was not to hurt her. But if she is hurt, you have to acknowledge your role in that. One of the secrets of mature friendship is sacrifice. Not blind, senseless sacrifice, but sacrifice for someone, for something—for your friendship. If she's hurt, that's what matters. Occasionally, you have to put her feelings first. Hopefully one day she'll do the same for you. Ask yourself: What's it really going to cost you to say you're sorry? Is it that big a deal?

What's important is that your friend is hurting. If you're ready to resolve things, find her. Do not talk to anyone else about it. Do not get "advice." Do not talk to her friends. Just find her and get her alone. Tell her you want to talk. Use some of the questions on page 53 to guide you. Then apologize.

Interviews with hundreds of girls had a major impact on my own friendships. I realized the girls' fears of direct conflict were no different than my own. After a lot of effort and reflection, I learned that what feels the hardest in a friendship often turns out, with practice, to be pretty easy, especially saying you're sorry. I used to anticipate major disasters if I took responsibility for my mistakes. Why would anyone want to be my friend if I had done something really wrong? Amazingly, I found that most people apologized right back. Once I opened the door with my apology, I was almost always met halfway.

Owning Up

In *Odd Girl Out,* I wrote about bullying my friend Anne in ninth grade. When Anne and I met ten years later to talk about it, she helped me realize that I had been in denial about the terrible things I had done. I lied to myself and others about who I was: the kind of person who would never do such a mean thing.

Of course, Anne had never forgotten. She described in precise detail what our group of friends had done to her, especially the effect it had had on her self-esteem. When I listened to her and then apologized, I believe I was able to give her some measure of peace, even a decade later.

If you have done something you regret, it is never too late to make amends. Hurting someone doesn't make you a terrible person. Nobody, none of us, is nice all the time and to everyone. *We all make mistakes.* You can still be a good person even if you have done some bad things. I think of myself that way, and I hope other girls will, too. Telling the truth about the darker sides of being a girl is actually an important thing to do—an act of girl power. When you take responsibility for the things you've done wrong and still work at being a good person, you help show the world that the nicest girls are actually real, flawed people, not perfect plastic dolls.

No matter how long ago it happened, you can always say you're sorry. Apologies never expire. You'll get a lot in return: You will walk away understanding yourself better and letting go of the secrets and shame so many girls are forced to hide. You'll find it easier to apologize in the everyday conflicts that arise in your life. Best of all, you will become a truer, more honest person in the process.

"I WANTED TO FIT IN SO BADLY"

Life as the Odd Girl Out

The letters in this section were the hardest for me to read. Their authors sounded like solitary, embattled soldiers in a terrible kind of war: one that never ended, pitted whole armies against them, and gave them no ammunition with which to fight back.

These writers bear the sad distinction of living for years in social exile. Often lacking the security of close, trusting friendships, they had no places to sleep over on the weekends, dates to meet people at the mall, guys to dance with at parties, or parties to go to at all. They were picked last for teams and had no one to talk with at lunch, in the halls, or at their lockers.

When I put myself in their shoes and try to imagine a life like that, I can hardly breathe. I realize how much I took the privileges of inclusion for granted. And I wonder if, years ago, I made an odd girl out feel more hopeless, more afraid, more alone.

Yet these stories call as much attention to the girls' extraordinary resilience as they do to the darkness of the human spirit. While so many girls grow up taking shelter in their friends, the storm of peer cruelty forces some girls to seek refuge in themselves. Face-to-face with hate, they somehow manage to become extraordinary young women: streetwise, cautious, kind, empathetic, and smart. I am awed by their courageous self-respect in the face of seemingly endless sorrow. Here are some of their stories.

I Wanted to Fit In So Badly

All of my life, I have never really, truly "fit in." I was never really part of a group. My family never really had the money to buy me all of the clothing that was "in style." However, I still managed and I loved my school. At the end of sixth grade it closed, forcing me to go to another school, to make another desperate attempt to "fit in."

I was the only new girl to come to seventh grade at school. There were about eleven or twelve of us seventh grade girls including me, and they were in two cliques. There were three really popular girls, and the semi-popular girls were all the rest. Our class was a mixture of both eighth graders and seventh graders, which made it even tougher because all the girls in eighth grade saw me as a loser, too.

Brittany, who was very popular and pretty, drew a picture when a substitute was in. It was a picture of the substitute naked, and she was quick to show the teacher and say that I drew it. I always got into trouble for pitiful little things such as these. I was an over-weight girl, very shy and timid.

Things never got really bad until eighth grade. I suffered all of the time. All of the other girls had numerous boyfriends. They talked about all the sexual things that they had done with them. I had never been with a boy, had a boyfriend, or even considered having one. I was never invited to the birthday parties or the little girl get-togethers they would have every other day.

I was teased about everything: my clothes, my hair, my weight, my long face, the fact that I had no boobs. Often I would just go home and cry. It seemed like the only way to ease the pain. I considered suicide but never actually went through with it.

It was between these tough times that my mother and I had gotten very close. We became like the best of friends. While I was dealing with all of the torment and taunting, I was having problems with my teacher. So I went to school and came home every day crying about how so-and-so had said this, and how I thought this so-and-so was my best friend, how could they betray me like that?

All of this teasing that I had already gone through was nothing compared to what was to come. I remember being at school in the computer lab one day, and this guy Nick asked me if I had said something about my cousin and how she had fucked her boyfriend or something. I responded no.

Later on that week, the girls from my class wanted

me to go to a dance. I found this odd, considering they never wanted me to do anything with them or even be near them. However, I said "okay." I wanted to fit in so badly. I didn't care.

Later on that night, I went into my closet and dug out my size thirteen formfitting jeans. I put them on and watched as my flab tumbled over the top of them. I put on my playgirl sweater, went into the bathroom, and put on some heavy makeup. I looked like a fat slut, but I didn't see it.

When I walked out of the bathroom, my mother told me to take off those jeans and go put on my windbreakers. She could see that it wasn't me. I never did like the tight formfitting clothes. However, I got pissed off at her and refused to talk to her, I was so bent on going to this dance and looking good.

It even got to the point where she told me that she would not allow me to leave the house until I at least changed my pants. When we began to leave and go to the dance, she dropped me off in front of the hall. I got out, still refusing to talk to her, and she said, "Call me if you want to leave earlier, I love you." Still I did not answer her. I quickly went inside and found all of the girls whom I had considered to be my friends standing there.

They all embraced me saying, "Hey there, I'm so happy that you could come." Moments afterward, a girl named Marie and my cousin confronted me.

Marie began to swear and curse at me saying things like, "You fucking fat bitch! Starting shit 'bout ma girl Randi here!" She went on forever, and not one person, not one, helped me. I stood there on the verge of tears, not saying anything, feeling betrayed and angered. Marie threatened me a few times and then walked away saying she was going to get her friends to kick my ass.

At that moment, I ran, scared shitless of what they might do to me, knowing that no one was ever going to help me. I ran out of the dance hall crying, I ran a long dark mile. I got to the nearest country-style donut shop where I knew some people. I went to a pay phone, called my mom, and broke down into tears. My mom quickly came and got me. I embraced her, shaking, terrified, and crying so hard that I was barely even able to get the words out of my mouth. She hugged me and we sat there in that parking lot for an hour.

We came home, and my mom called my cousin's mother. She instantly began to side with Randi, saying that I had always been backward and blah blah blah. Randi had done nothing, all that her mom could see was her sweet little angel who she let do whatever the hell she wanted to.

The next day I went to school, and as I walked in, I was told by one of the popular girls to "leave, like seriously, just die." I thought she was joking, as she was known as the drama queen, so I laughed. But then when everyone was staring at me I realized, Oh my god, she's serious. I ran inside and cried again.

I made myself sick in the bathroom so that I could come home. Once I told my mom, she kept me home from school for a week. When I went back I got the same looks and curses from the same people. I was an outcast, and everyone around our little town knew my name, for a bad reason. A majority wanted to kick my ass.

I began to feel really insecure about myself. I went on a diet thinking, maybe if I'm thin they will like me. I began losing weight, first twenty pounds, then thirty pounds. By graduation, I had gone down from a size thirteen to a nine. I was very proud of myself. I had gone from 178 pounds and 5' 5" to 148 pounds.

The others around me continued to be unimpressed. Since the rumors, I hadn't talked to anyone. I would not leave my house or talk on the phone. I was scared. After school was over, I was so happy. I lost more weight in the summer and I grew, too. By the end of the summer, I was around 5' 7" and 121 pounds. When I went back to my dietitian, she said that this was unhealthy, and that I needed to stop dieting because I was very underweight. She gave me exercises to do so that I might be able to build some muscle.

Now I sit at a happy 142 pounds. My friends tell me I look great, and I do feel it. I'm so proud of myself. I have true friends now that I just couldn't bear to live without. They keep me going. They are a big part of me and who I am. My marks are doing fine. I still don't have a boyfriend, but I really don't have the desire to have one anymore. Since I go to high school in another town, I stay with my new friends as much as possible.

I am still scared of my hometown and the people in it. But I have left them behind because they don't matter anymore. I'm me. I'm not tiny, I'm not the most beautiful person in the world, but I'm me and that's all that I can be. And even though the past will continue to haunt me and will scar me for life, I know in my heart my friends will always be there to help me through it. I can't believe it. Oh my god, I have friends.

—AGE 18

I Am Me

I was one of those little kids that would just make you melt. I was an Asian mother's dream: beautiful, smart, perfect grades, articulate, respectful, and happy. I played more with guys than girls because my neighborhood was packed with boys and I got tired of making daisy links and Barbies. Girls were boring in my opinion.

I loved school. I never had trouble with it because I was liked and I was the smartest one in the class. I never got anything lower than an A–, and I hated that minus sign.

In third grade, I moved to a new elementary school. Naturally, I hung out with the Asian girls. I made friends quickly. But one girl named Karen apparently didn't like me hanging out with *her* friends. She gave me dirty looks and eventually started spreading rumors about me. I never got to know what they were.

The girls whispered in secret, they stared at me with slitty eyes that made your skin crawl, and they excluded me from everything. I was always the last one picked.

Soon, all the Asian girls started hating me. I was hurt because I usually got the most attention. I had never been so put down in my life, and things only got worse. The non-Asian girls hated me, too. The guys, of course, joined in the whole teasing thing. By the end of the school year, I was totally alone and hurt. In fourth grade, nothing got better.

I started to hate school and told my mother. My mom got angry and said that I was just being a bad girl. She said that people can't possibly hate you unless you did something heinously wrong. She wouldn't listen, so I gave up talking about school. I tried everything to be nice to Karen and her friends. I even nominated Karen for class president and all their jaws dropped. She was nice to me for some time, but then she got angry when I got a better grade on something. I was alone again. I eventually started hating her.

Her mother came to me and told *me* to stop hurting *Karen.* In what way? I asked. You ask her what *she's* doing to *me.* Her mom looked like she was going to slap me. I wondered what loads of lies Karen had told her mother. I couldn't beat her up because the wimp always kept many friends around. Besides, I'd be a bad girl if I hit someone; it was a lesson taught to me since I could remember.

By the end of fourth grade, I had grown a shell to hide all my emotions and thoughts. If I had backed down and been a follower type of girl, perhaps she would've stopped. But no, I always had something to say back. That really drove her insane. I would never back down because I had pride.

I was also practically the only Korean girl there. They were all Chinese, Malaysian, Taiwanese, or some other Asian type. I became racist, too, thinking that only Koreans were worthy Asians and the others were smelly trash that deserved to die. In my eyes, such hate could not come from normal people. I still remember them giggling, passing notes, glaring, and fighting over who had to have me on their team.

I was just plain old Anna. The only thing they respected was my knowledge. On our end-of-the-year project, they wrote: creative, smart, nice, friendly, good at spelling, and stuff like that. If they knew this, why were they so mean to me? I didn't understand it, and it drove me insane.

In fifth grade, I was a mental wreck. I cried every day. The only other Korean kid was a girl who stopped being my friend and made me look bad in front of my mom. My mom didn't believe a *child* could be so "stressed" and only told me to shut up.

You know how kids travel in groups? Well, when one got kicked out, she'd come to me. We would be the nicest friends until she stabbed me in the back when she got back to her group. She'd act like she never knew me.

I decided to kill myself and stared at the concrete

wall. I was crying, afraid, but right before I was going to ram my head into it, a couple of boys came and started to tease me. I cried and realized I was afraid to die. So I couldn't end my misery either way. My teacher, Mr. Cusack, told me I had "emotional" problems and was a social "disaster." He never took my side. He made me teach other stupid kids who couldn't figure out their fractions.

Tom, Karen's brother, was in my class that year. One day we had a bitter fight, and he made Tom apologize. Mr. Cusack dragged Tom and me to the front of the room. Tom got to sit down, but I was up in the front of the classroom while Mr. Cusack talked about me and loners. He asked the class to be nice and pity me. He said it'd be hard but to try their best. They nodded and all looked at me. They snickered and said, "We have to be nice to you now, don't we?"

I learned how to be angry, bitter, and talk back. Even though I looked so strong inside, I trembled. Inside, I wanted to die, but I'd never show them that. I learned how to become a bitch. I totally changed into a person with split personalities. One was this sweet, nice, smart, talkative, and happy child. Another was a depressed, bitchy, sad, suicidal, mute, and stunned girl.

In sixth grade, I thought everything would be better, because two other schools were coming along with mine to middle school. But nothing got better. Padma, an ugly, stupid, loner girl kept hanging around my group. I was friends with the seventh graders (the "sevvys," as we called them). Everyone talked about how I was best friends with Padma. I wasn't her friend! I hated her! She not only was smelly, ugly, and mean, but she was selfish, gross, spiteful, and an all-around rotten person.

I joined drama club and got the lead role as the queen. I loved acting and I was the star. I met my best friends Jennifer and Callie there. Drama was my special thing that kept me happy. Jennifer and Callie told me I was the nicest girl. They said that they didn't understand how anyone could be so mean to me.

In the seventh grade, people knew about my "reputation" and they were meaner than hell. I expected an insult every period.

In the locker room, a girl I didn't even know asked me, "Are you Anna?" I said yes. "You're a bitch!" she said, and giggled and walked off.

I saw my counselor every Wednesday. I told her everything. She just nodded and listened, and I just rattled on. What frustrated me most was that she didn't *do* anything. She just gave me "uh-huhs," said "I see..." and "I'm sorry, dear." I became frustrated and stopped going altogether.

I finally got so fed up that I wrote Karen a note saying that I wanted to talk to her with the mediators at school. She freaked out because she was Miss Goody Two-Shoes and had never been in trouble in her life. To prevent anything from happening, she wrote me back.

She said, "I'm really sorry. I was too embarrassed to

apologize in front of my friends. I don't even really know why I did it. Please forgive me. Oh, and can we please not go to the counselor? I'd prefer not to."

I finally realized that I hadn't done anything wrong. She was just stupid and jealous and wanted to make my life miserable. But the damage was done. It wasn't her group that bothered me anymore; it was the big huge group of people at school. What she started couldn't be reversed.

On the very last day of school, Padma came up to me. We had the same P.E. class.

"You *bitch*! You slut! I hate you!" she spurted.

I got really pissed and I glared (something I learned from Karen) and said, "What are you talking about? I've *never* been mean to you!"

"You made Callie not be friends with me anymore! I hate you!" she was sobbing her ugly heart out.

Brianna and Sophie were also in my P.E. class. They were eighth graders now, and I was really close to them. They said, "Well, she *is* the quiet one. Gawd, Anna, why are you so mean? Come, Padma, we'll let you wash up and talk, okay?" Then they left. I was so utterly shocked, I couldn't speak.

I hung out with my drama friends and all the other loser leftover people. I was okay with a few of them, but I hated the rest. They were the lowest of the low. I cried a lot because every day something would happen. I was so strong before, but it was impossible now. Think about it. A bad day can pass. A bad week is just a bummer week. A month makes you crabby, but not broken. A year starts to deteriorate you. But six years can kill you.

I went on the Washington, D.C., trip with Callie. A curious popular girl asked me why people hated me so much. I told her my story. She nodded and sorted it out so that the popular kids wouldn't be as harsh as before. I hung out with them. They liked me. I felt awesome. I felt like I was at the top of the world.

When we got back, Callie avoided me. She wouldn't talk, and most of all, she stopped waiting for me to go to classes. I asked her what was wrong, and she said that some girl told her that I had never been her friend and I only put up with her because I felt like it. I told her I never said that, but after that, Callie always ignored me. My own best friend ignored me.

We had gone to the knowledge competition the year before. Callie, Christina, Jennifer, and I were in one group. I thought we were in the same group for sure that year, and I said that. She only nodded slightly.

I found out that she kicked me out and put Kai in the group instead. Reynu told me that and she said, "Uh, yeah, you're sort of not in the group, so just find another one." I was devastated to find Callie, Christina, and Kai talking like old friends, like how they used to talk to me. I was at the exact same table and I cried. They didn't even notice.

Jennifer did. Jennifer was angry because she was never told. She bailed out. I thought maybe if Jennifer left, Callie would definitely ask me back. But even if she did ask me, I wouldn't go because that would be using Jennifer. I waited for her to ask. She didn't. In fact, she asked a girl she barely even knew to join. I was so hurt because by choosing a girl she didn't even know she was saying that our friendship didn't mean anything to her.

At the end of the school year, none of them wanted me around. They backstabbed me and didn't even care about me. Jennifer was the only one that stuck by me.

I repeatedly thought about killing myself. All the while, my parents couldn't figure out why I was stressed out, why I came home drying tears, and why I was so changed. My mother and father fought all the time. I didn't know what was worse, school or home.

Now that I look back, I remember that I was mean to a few people. I totally shunned Padma after she called me a bitch. I went along with the rumors. I even told the other kids about how she picked at her wedgies onstage, how she picked her boogers, how she smelled, and all the other usual junk we talked about. I gave her the leering looks, talked behind her back, and all the other things. I felt good because she was lower than even me, and because I wanted her to feel the pain I felt. I wish I had never done it now. It's wrong, and nobody really cared.

I go to a wonderful school now. I'm deathly scared of going to the public high school because that's where all of them are. Going through the emotional trauma would kill me. I now realize that I'm not a fat, ugly, mean, and all-around bitch. I was a victim like so many others. It takes a while to get used to people telling me that I'm pretty, skinny, and the nicest person they know. It makes me feel all confused. But I don't care about popularity anymore. I realized that I'm special, that people like me for who I am here. And I will never try to become another person again.

—AGE 15

FINDING YOUR INNER STRENGTH

Some people's struggles to fit in at school never end. Year by year, they make and lose friends, get bullied, and suffer heartache. No one really knows for sure why some kids are rejected repeatedly. As I showed in *Odd Girl Out,* it's not just the poor, overweight, or weird girls who are targets. It could be anyone.

What's amazing to me is not how many girls suffer, but how many triumph over their ordeals. Girls who are humiliated and demeaned, who are abused physically and emotionally, who don't want to come to school, who have thought about dying, find extraordinary inner strength. They learn from their perpetrators who they don't want to be, and in their frequent isolation, figure out exactly who they are and what they want. These girls are role models for me, and their stories can be found throughout this book, especially before and after this section.

If you are the odd girl out more often than not, please read the advice I give to girls on pages 101–03 (in When Friends Turn On You). Beyond that, I suggest the following:

- Ask your parents about visiting a psychotherapist. I saw one when I was a teenager, and she made a huge difference in my life. A good therapist won't judge you; she'll be on your side and help you get through difficult times. If it's appropriate, she'll steer you into social skills training or help you with it directly.

- Find your voice and use it. Work with a therapist, counselor, or parent on saying "no," or "stop," to the people who are trying to ruin your life. Role play the conversations, or study theater to practice using your voice. Take karate, tae kwon do, or kickboxing; they connect you with the physical power of your body and boost your self-esteem. Harness your power and challenge yourself to fight back. Stand up and say what you want and what you don't, and if you can't get it by asking firmly, seek out other ways.

- Get involved—really involved—in activities outside of school. Find something to fall for, and let your passion for it distract you. When I was a teenager and I felt like no person understood me, I spent hours every week with horses. When I couldn't stand my own life, I read, and disappeared into someone else's. I also loved basketball. I could stamp out all thoughts except getting that ball in the basket.

- As my mom always says, living well is the best revenge. So live well: Create a life for yourself outside the sphere of your troubles. As you probably know, one of the worst things about being rejected is the feeling that the pain will never end. When you meet people who have no connection to your social misfortune, you can inhabit another world. When you find something to do that will introduce you to new friends, the positive relationships you'll forge will be your best evidence that this won't always be your life. And if you can find just one friend, he or she could buffer you against the torment you're facing. One friend can be shelter from the storm.

- If you're feeling depressed—eating less or more, sleeping less or more, hating or considering harming yourself—get help. Call 1-800-SUICIDE (784-2433) for immediate support by telephone, or visit www.teenadviceonline.org to chat with a counselor, ask a question, or read about depression. No one should have to go through this alone.

If you can do nothing else, just remember: It will end. You will move on. You will not always be at this school, in that bed, with these parents. Life is long, and you are stronger than you think.

Why Are We So Cruel?

A different kind of battle
There is no ammunition
No blood to prove its existence
No physical impairment at all
But it's there...
An invisible battle
Utter stillness, silence
No one speaks
No one acknowledges.
In tight packs they stay close
With their hair all intertwined in a line
Alliances... defined:
Once outside, the doors instantly lock
But no one sees
The invisible battle.
Squinted eyes of hatred pierce a heart
But I can't dress the wound
Why can't I just swing my arm?
Patch up my body
And go on.

Stereotypically we're dainty, passive,
Everything must be indiscernible
Until preoccupation swells
Funneling every ounce of energy into a hollow
    opening
To think about the painful obsession
Of the now massively dramatized enemy:
Us

                                              —AGE 17

I Was the One Word that Everyone Fears: Alone

Have you ever heard the phrase, "What goes around, comes around"? Or even, "If you do something bad, it will come back to you three times worse"? I never believed these myths until they actually happened to me. Having to maintain a certain image of perfection, my town isn't always considered the friendliest. The people are uptight and sometimes a little bit hard to handle. Even though I have grown up there, the people still shock me, and so do their children.

In second grade I transferred to a small private school down the road from my house. I have always been open and easy to talk to, so making new friends wasn't a problem for me. I became best friends with a group of girls. We were inseparable and did everything together. We did everything from sharing our "deepest darkest secrets" to talking about what we want to be when we grow up to making fun of nearly all the kids not involved in our clique.

We were considered the "popular" group. We intimidated everyone and it seemed that everyone knew that but me. I was just going on with my little fourth grade life and having fun. Now that I look back on what I was like in second, third, fourth, and fifth grade, I can call myself a bitch. Like all my friends, I was nice to everyone's faces and then talked horribly behind their backs. Because I was so young, I didn't know that what I was doing was wrong and kept doing it until I had it done back to me.

Boys were beginning to become a huge thing in fourth and fifth grade. Sometimes a girl had her status by the boy she dated, so naturally every girl wanted the "Most Popular Boy in the Grade." In fifth grade, I was going out with a boy named Luke who everyone thought was perfect. The competition for him was gleaming and the jealousy for him was outrageous.

I had no idea that my friends were talking behind my back about how I "don't deserve him" and "Ugh, he deserves SO much better than her . . . someone like me!" When I finally found out what my friends were saying about me, it was worse than a slap in the face.

It was a Sunday morning and my phone rang at 8:30. I picked up the phone to my best friend, Rachel, who I trusted with my life.

"Hi, Grace. I just got an e-mail from Luke saying that he dumped you for me. Umm . . . so, what's up?"

"What?" I said, "I don't understand, he hasn't dumped me. Hold on, let me check my e-mail." Sure enough, I had received an e-mail from Luke with the subject of "Good-bye." He had dumped *me* for *Rachel*?

What? My fifth grade ego completely popped right there and then. I was astonished. I didn't know what to do. The following week was hard but not even close to what was going to come.

I lowered my head every time I passed Luke and his posse to avoid their looks. It's all right, I thought, at least I still have my girlfriends.

I noticed some minor differences with my friends. They seemed to be ignoring me more lately. I thought that it might be the small side effects of my breakup with Luke, but I was very wrong.

I came home from school that week in the middle of April and checked my e-mail. (I seemed to have lived on e-mail in fifth grade!) I opened up a letter from Rachel and tears started to stream down my face as I read on. Sentences like, "You make my life a living hell," and "Frankly, if you switched schools, people would either be happy or couldn't care less. Sadly, I'd be both," made the tears just flow harder. She was my best friend. How could she do this to me? She had even said that the other girls hated me.

Why? What had I ever done to them? I had done nothing.

The next months at school were ridiculous. I called my mom crying every day at recess time begging her to come pick me up. She refused and said that she believed in me and that I could get through this. Each day, the comments and the stares got worse and worse. When I walked into a room, they would all say something like,

"Shh!! She's coming!! Ugh, I guess we might *have* to be quiet or else she'll go and tell her friends. Oh wait! She doesn't have any!"

It was true, though; I had no friends. The ones I had trusted had abandoned me, and I was left with the people who I made fun of. I didn't know what to do. I was the one word that everyone fears: alone.

One day at sports the girls in the grade were playing a game of Capture the Flag. This girl, Tara, who seemed to get pleasure out of making my life a nightmare, was talking to her friend and pointing at me. I went up to her (she was on the opposing team, and standing right on the edge of the line that separates the teams), and I said, "Do you have a problem with me? What did I *ever* do to you? *Nothing!* That's right, I didn't do anything. You're just making fun of me because you're a follower and have nothing better to do with your life."

That pushed her over the edge. She took my arm, pulled me onto her side, and slapped me. I was astonished and just started to cry. The teacher came. She gathered the girls into a huge group and told them that if they weren't nice to me, then the school would have to take action. She threatened them with suspension.

Throughout the rest of fifth grade and during sixth, I made amazing friends. These girls were awesome. In the previous years I was too caught up with making fun of these girls to see how incredible they were. Although the girls who ridiculed me apologized, I never became too close to them, which was the mistake I had made before.

In seventh and eighth grade I became friends with everyone. I was the only girl who was not subscribed to a certain clique or group. The guys in my grade were always so laid back and chill that I decided to start hanging out with them. Before you knew it, I had the best friends you could ever ask for. Through my experiences, I became a stronger person. I learned so much about myself and about others. Because of what happened, I am more confident and happy with myself. There is no way I would be the same person I am today if I hadn't gone through the torture I went through in fifth grade.

When I told my friends that I was going to an all-girls' school, they were all shocked. "Grace? Going to an *all-girls' school*? What is going through her head?" I can admit that before I came to my school, I was nervous about the girls and what the whole scenario was going to be like. The moment I stepped out of the car on the first day, I loved it. Of course everyone has their closest friends, but there are no cliques or "popular" and "unpopular" girls. Everyone seems equal. At my new school, the realization of girl friendships has embraced me.

—AGE 15

Happy

Happy is a state of mind. I once thought that I was happy, and I wasn't. I didn't even know the meaning of happy. But I now know the true meaning of the word, and I've found happiness inside of me. All three of my middle school years were spent trying to make myself and others believe that I was happy. It took me a year to realize that I wasn't happy, that I was only faking. I then spent another year and a half trying to do everything I could to make myself happy, and truly believe and feel happy. When in fact I had no idea what real happiness was.

In middle school, I always felt as if I was an "odd girl out" because I never really had one certain group of friends like most of the people I know. Most of the African American "cliques" said I acted and talked too much like a "white girl." I wasn't "black" enough to hang out with them. To this group of people I became known as the "smart, happy, black cheerleader who acts like a white girl." My answer to that is . . . why? Is it because I speak proper English, I make good grades, I walk around with a smile on my face and my head held high? If that was why, then so what? That's just me. I was generally a happy person, or at least I thought I was. I would walk around perky, and always with a smile on my face.

That's another thing I think African American girls didn't like about me, my sense of happiness. One girl even told me that she had never met a black girl who was always happy and had a smile on her face. To me, that was a compliment. I never thought much about it. It was just who I was. I never had a problem with hanging out with Caucasian girls, but it just seemed that I couldn't find that right social group that I could be a part of.

At one point I thought I had found a group of friends that I could join. It was an ethnically mixed group of girls that at first treated me great. I soon learned that they had a sort of "leader," who I became very close to. I soon saw her true colors when I realized that she was using me, and became very disrespectful toward my family and me. I stayed for a while and put up with the disrespect; don't ask me why. I guess I was so happy about feeling like I belonged, I didn't care what she said or did. Eventually, I got tired of it, so I left. I continue to be friends with some of the girls, but it's not like it used to be.

While all of this was going on at school, I also had a ton of family issues to deal with. My parents were on the verge of separation. The fighting, harsh words, and coming home to just one parent each night was a lot to grasp. I know you may be thinking that it's not uncommon, but for someone who has had both parents every day ever since they were born, it's hard. The transformations going on inside our home were huge, and I had to deal with them alone. I had to deal with the tears alone because I felt that I had no one to talk to. My parents weren't around, and when they were, they were either arguing or upset.

Well, ya know, when it rains, it pours. Just as all of this was erupting in my life, I began to have issues with me. I began to look at myself and compare myself to others. Physically, I wasn't satisfied with what I saw in the mirror. There were times when I didn't eat and would do everything I could to avoid eating. This became an obsession, which quickly made me very weak and very sick.

No one at home noticed because they had their own problems to deal with. Mentally, I began to wonder what was wrong with me, and why I couldn't have friends like everyone else. I began looking for ways to change my personality. My focus became transforming myself into what others wanted me to be. I tried it, and I hated the new me, worse than the old me. So I gave up on changing, believing that I would never have friends.

In the midst of all of this, I was still at school walking around with a smile on my face, pretending that nothing was wrong. It soon caught up with me, and I realized that all this time I had been faking my happiness. I hid my tears behind my fake smiles and fake laughs so that no one would notice. I had forgotten how to really smile and really laugh, but I knew I wanted to remember. No one knew this, and I had been trying to cover it up. I couldn't do it anymore.

I began to search for my happiness. Keep in mind that I'm one of those independent-for-life types and I don't (if I can help it) depend on anybody for anything. I began to turn to people for happiness, and I would become frustrated when it didn't work or they didn't make me happy. I began to turn to things that I generally would never turn to. I turned to food, which comforted me but had bad repercussions. When I turned to television, it only reminded me of the things that I longed for, including the happiness that I felt I would never find.

I began to write poetry to express my feelings; it allowed me write down the things that were upsetting me, but let's face it, paper doesn't talk back. None of these things worked. I might want to mention that I'm also a single-for-life type, and at one point I thought that turning to a boyfriend would help. This idea was sparked by my observance of my peers and their courtships. They looked extremely happy and told me how happy they were when they were with their boyfriends. Okay, I didn't go that far, but I was close. I contemplated it many times, but I didn't really believe that was what I was looking for.

It was then that I realized that what I wanted was

someone to talk to, I wanted someone to listen to me. The one thing that I turned to that helped me greatly was music. I could always find a song with lyrics that expressed what I was feeling and still do today. Music comforted me unlike anything I had ever tried.

I've learned that God will show up in your life when you least expect it. I know he did in mine. I came home one night, alone, after a bad day. I walked into the bathroom, took one look at my sad face in the mirror, and I knew I couldn't hold the pain in any longer. I took another look at myself, and I broke down and cried. As I cried, I began to think about where I was the last time I was truly happy.

It occurred to me that the last time I had been truly happy was when I was in church. The happy spirits, inspirational music, and the all-around happy sensation that I felt always seemed to uplift my spirit. Now, I wasn't brought up going to church every Sunday, or even every other Sunday, so it had really been a while since I'd been to church.

I began to recollect on some of the sermons that I had listened to in the past, but had never actually taken the time to comprehend and apply them to my life. One of the sermons that I remembered was a sermon on the power of prayer. This sermon spoke on how effective and truly amazing the power of prayer is.

I had heard stories about people praying to God for his blessings and forgiveness, and also how he answers all prayers. Prayer in my life had never been completely imperative, nor at times realistic. Every once in a while I prayed over meals, but only because someone told me to; to me it was just a hassle. I had never prayed on my own free will. I never saw the point.

At that moment, I dropped to my knees and I prayed. I prayed for all of the things in my life that I felt kept me from my happiness. I prayed for my parents, I prayed for friendship, I prayed for love, self-love, and self-acceptance, but most of all, I prayed for happiness.

After my prayer, I turned on my radio, and Yolanda Adams's "Open My Heart" was on. I was bawling again. The song touched me, and I knew at that moment I needed God in my life. I knew that I wanted to give my life to Christ. I didn't know it at the time, but at that moment, God spoke to me. He told me that he would be my friend, he would wipe my tears, he would soothe my pain, he would never leave me, and most importantly, he would love me unconditionally. All I had to do was believe.

Ever since that night, my whole outlook on life has changed. The moment I accepted God into my life and my heart, I found my happiness. God shined his light in places in my life that I thought would be dark forever. He's taken away all of my pain and replaced it with joy and love. I'm not saying that I'll never hurt, and I'll never have problems. Who doesn't? It's now, through him, that I've learned how to deal with my problems in a positive way, through prayer, and with faith that everything will turn out right.

I've found that happiness is not something that is easily gained. It's something that comes deep within yourself. It's something that I believe is a blessing from God. To be truly happy, I believe that you have to learn to love and accept yourself for who and what you are, even if no one else does. God loves you, and his love is all that you'll ever need.

I encourage you today to take a look at your inner self. Are you truly happy? If not, take a look at your spirituality, and through it, look to discover your inner happiness. I found my happiness in God, and in my happiness, I've found the acceptance and love that I have been searching for.

So now, when people ask me why I'm so happy and why I'm always smiling, I put on a bright smile and say: "God is good!" I don't have a reason not to smile, because God has truly smiled on me.

—AGE 14

I'm Not Out, But I'm Still Not In

My neighborhood wasn't the poor type, but it wasn't really rich either. However, there was still enough money to go around, and we lived in one of the wealthiest counties in the United States. My elementary school was in the same county. Through my years there, plenty of new students entered the school, but by fifth grade, we all knew each other and were like a big family. Everyone knew each other, was friends, helped each other out, and that year was my greatest year of all.

I was the only one from my class in the Academically Talented program, better known as AT; I had the top grades in my class, my tests and quizzes were always the highest, and my friends and I developed an even tighter relationship than we'd ever had. I felt so good about myself.

Things went great until we started middle school. There were other kids that joined me in AT who seemed smarter than me, so I didn't feel so smart anymore. My tests and grades were still high, but I wasn't the only one with them. There were other kids getting the same grades as me, sometimes even better than mine.

But the worst thing that happened was that my friends left me for other people, new people that had come from other elementary schools. I often blame myself for that awful change. We were in classes depending on our level of capability and achievement, and coming from a lower-class school, most of my friends were in the lesser-regarded classes. They were all in the "low classes." That was how the smarter people referred to them.

Since we were all now in different classes, I didn't feel like part of their big, friendly family anymore. . . . I was the only one from my elementary school in the higher classes. The other girls in AT were all best friends already, so they seemed perfectly content. They were pretty, popular, smart, friendly, flirtatious, and almost everything else that I wasn't.

Despite their rare attempts to become my friend, I didn't talk to them much. I excluded myself from them and the rest of the school. Instead, I focused my life on school, making my grades go higher, higher, and higher, until I was close enough to a perfect 4.0 to almost touch it.

That wasn't what I wanted. No matter how high my grades were, I was still lonely and sad. I hardly smiled anymore, and even my family noticed. If anyone ever asked "What's the matter?" the answer was always "I'm just tired." My parents began to monitor my sleep to make sure I was getting enough, which I was. I sank deeper and deeper into despair, until I realized I could sink no deeper.

I finally decided to do something. The next day, a few of the girls in my classes tried to talk to me. Instead of brushing them off, this time I actually talked back. We began to start an interesting conversation, and soon enough I was talking and laughing with them daily. At lunch, everyone wanted to sit at their table, but there were so many people that all of their friends combined had to sit at two separate tables close to each other.

One day I walked into the lunchroom, heading for my usual corner of the room to eat with the few friends that I had remaining from elementary. They hardly talked to me, but they had still been my friends at one point, so I felt fine. There was some small talk between us often, but other than that we didn't talk. I wasn't unwelcome, but I wasn't exactly greeted with open arms and smiling faces either.

I heard a few voices calling my name. I turned and saw that the girls from my AT class were calling me. It was a total shocker, but I recovered. I didn't talk much during the meal, but it was still fun to be absorbed in their conversation, feeling like I was part of something special. I even stood with them during recess. That was the start of our friendship.

One of the girls, I noticed, kept being pushed around. Not physically, but she was often excluded from the group, pushed away as if not wanted. I wasn't in the center circle of the group myself, so I decided to talk to her, make her see that we both had something in common when it came to this situation.

Sure enough we became best friends the rest of the year and the summer. The second year of middle school, I expected things to be pretty much the same. I was wrong again. The table was less crowded so I always sat with them at lunch, but they seemed to be more flirtatious this year, even my best friend. They kept a lot of secrets and personal jokes, and whenever I asked about it, the answer was always, "It's a long story." Well, most of the stories, jokes, and secrets didn't seem that long, because they had plenty of time to tell the other people.

I just let it go unnoticed. After all, I'd spent a whole year without any friends, so I could last this year without knowing some secrets. Well, things really got out of hand. There were too many secrets, and I wasn't sure if they were talking about me. I felt really uncomfortable, but I didn't have anywhere else to go. This was the only group of people that really accepted me, I think.

It lasted a whole year, and soon I even began to cry at night because I felt so left out. My best friend had joined them in the secrets, so I had no one to lean on. I felt like a single grain of sand in a desert going unnoticed because I was no different from the rest. Besides, if they were going to keep secrets from me, they could at least make it a little less obvious. They could be